TABLE OF CONTENTS

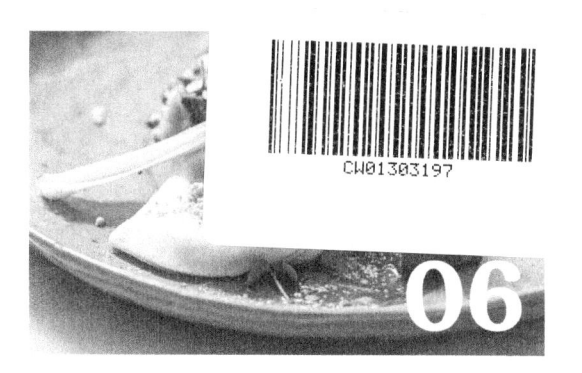

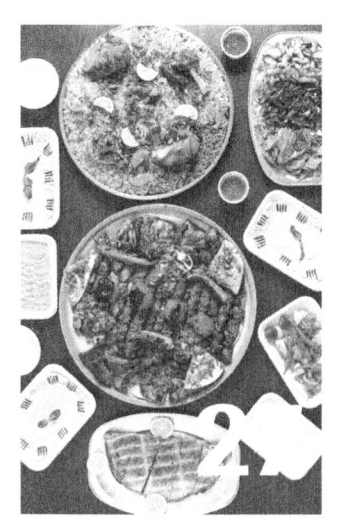

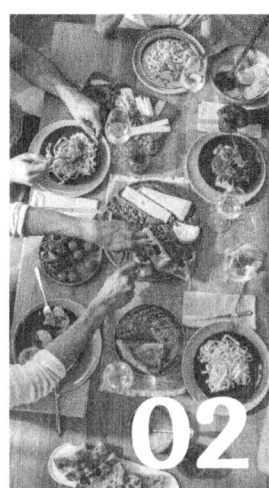

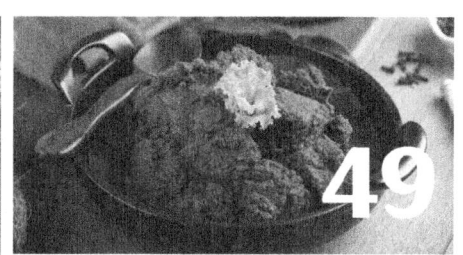

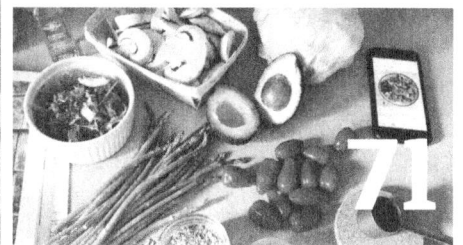

Introduction — 02

This part gives you a general idea about the contents of the book, how the weight watchers program work, and the benefits.

Chapter 1: Breakfast — 06

Chapter 1 provides 20 breakfast recipes

Chapter 2: Lunch — 27

Chapter 2 provides 20 lunch recipes

Chapter 3: Dinner — 49

Chapter 3 provides 30 dinner recipes

Chapter 4: Dessert — 71

Chapter 4 provides 10 dessert recipes

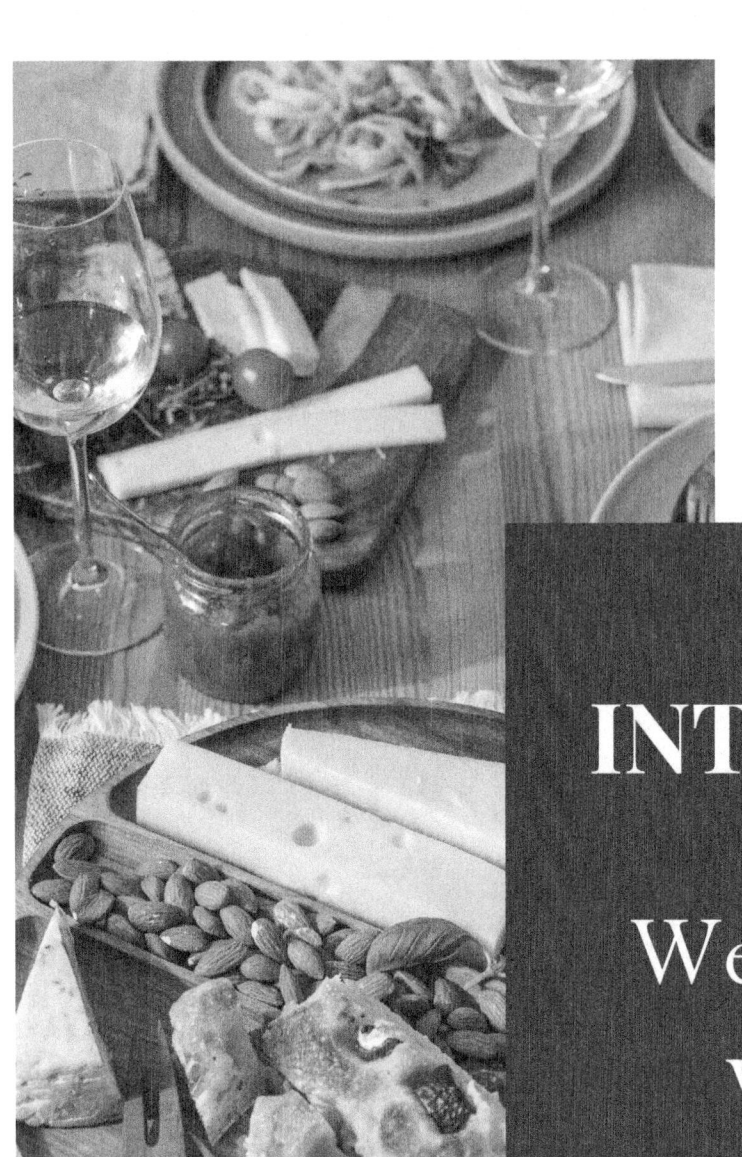

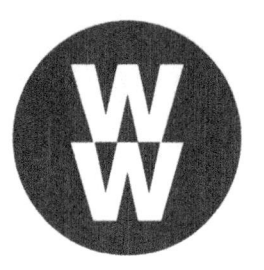

INTRODUCTION

Weight Watchers Weight Loss Program

01
Breakfast

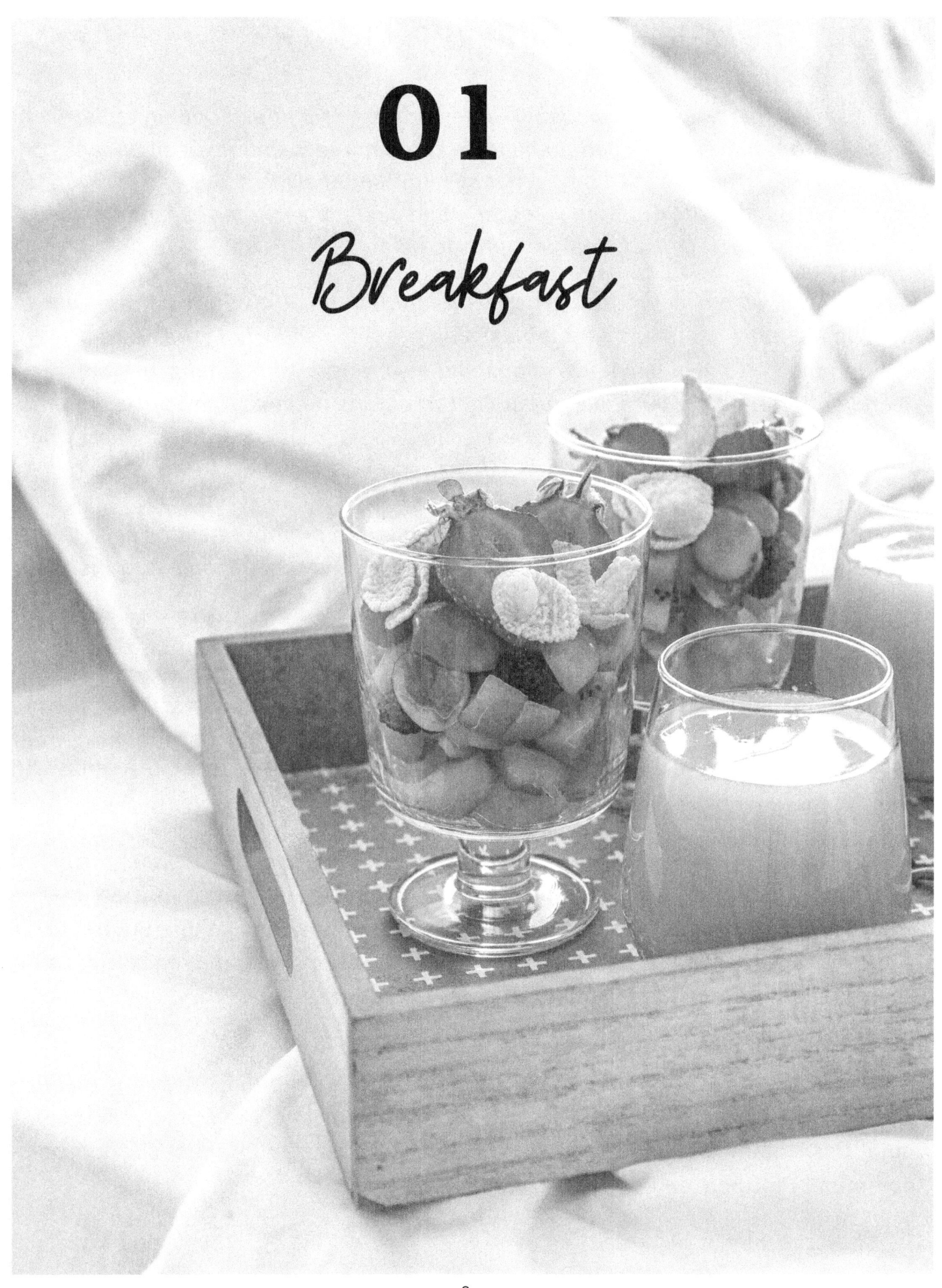

ABOUT THE WEIGHT WATCHERS PROGRAM

Weight Watchers, now known as WW International, is a popular commercial weight loss program that offers a comprehensive approach to weight loss and healthy living. The program is based on a point system that assigns a value to every food and drink based on its nutritional content, and assigns each participant a daily point goal based on their gender, age, weight, and height.

The program also encourages participants to adopt healthy eating habits, such as consuming more fruits and vegetables, lean proteins, and whole grains, while limiting their intake of unhealthy foods and beverages. Additionally, Weight Watchers offers a supportive community through its meetings and online forums, as well as personalized coaching and tracking tools to help participants stay on track with their weight loss goals.

Overall, the Weight Watchers program is designed to promote healthy and sustainable weight loss by helping individuals make gradual changes to their diet and lifestyle.

HOW DOES THE PROGRAM WORK?

The Weight Watchers program uses a point system called SmartPoints, which assigns a point value to every food and drink based on its nutritional content. Each participant is given a daily SmartPoints target, based on their gender, age, weight, and height, which they can use to track their food intake and stay within their calorie budget.

The SmartPoints system takes into account the protein, carbohydrates, fat, and fiber content of foods, as well as their calorie density and other factors. Foods that are high in protein and fiber, for example, have a lower SmartPoints value than foods that are high in sugar or saturated fat.

In addition to tracking food intake, Weight Watchers also encourages participants to adopt healthy habits such as regular exercise, drinking plenty of water, and getting enough sleep. The program provides tools and resources to help participants set and track their goals, such as a mobile app, online community forums, and personalized coaching.

Weight Watchers also offers in-person meetings where participants can connect with others who are also trying to lose weight and get support from trained coaches. There is also a virtual program available for those who prefer to participate online.

Overall, the Weight Watchers program aims to provide a holistic approach to weight loss and healthy living, by helping individuals make sustainable lifestyle changes that can improve their overall health and well-being.

WHAT BENEFITS DO WEIGHT WATCHERS DIETS BRING?

The benefits of Dr. Nowzaradan's weight loss program can be significant, particularly for people who are severely obese. Some of the potential benefits of the program include:

Weight loss

Research has found that individuals who follow the Weight Watchers program lose more weight than those who try to lose weight on their own or with other diets.

Personalized approach

The program takes into account an individual's unique needs and preferences, such as their age, weight, height, and activity level, and provides personalized recommendations and support.

Sustainable weight loss

The program is designed to promote gradual, sustainable weight loss by making healthy lifestyle changes that can be maintained long-term.

Supportive community

Weight Watchers offers a supportive community of fellow participants and trained coaches who can provide encouragement and motivation to help individuals reach their weight loss goals.

Improved overall health

The Weight Watchers program encourages participants to consume more fruits, vegetables, lean proteins, and whole grains, which can improve overall health by reducing the risk of chronic diseases such as heart disease, diabetes, and cancer.and enjoy a more active lifestyle.

Flexibilityawareness

The program allows participants to enjoy their favorite foods in moderation and encourages physical activity, making it a more sustainable approach to weight loss compared to restrictive diets.

GREEK YOGURT WITH FRESH FRUIT & ALMONDS 2

This Greek yogurt breakfast bowl is a satisfying and delicious way to start your day. It's packed with protein, fiber, and healthy fats, and can be customized with your favorite fruits and nuts.

Prep: 5 mins or less
Cooking: 5 mins
Serve: 01

INGREDIENTS

- 1/2 cup plain Greek yogurt: 0 SmartPoints
- 1/2 cup mixed fresh fruit (such as berries, chopped apple, or sliced banana): 0 SmartPoints
- 1 tablespoon slivered almonds: 2 SmartPoints

INSTRUCTIONS

1. Spoon the Greek yogurt into a breakfast bowl.
2. Top with the fresh fruit and slivered almonds.
3. Serve and enjoy!

NUTRITIONS

Approximate, based on using 1/2 cup of non-fat Greek yogurt, 1/2 cup of mixed berries, and 1 tablespoon of slivered almonds

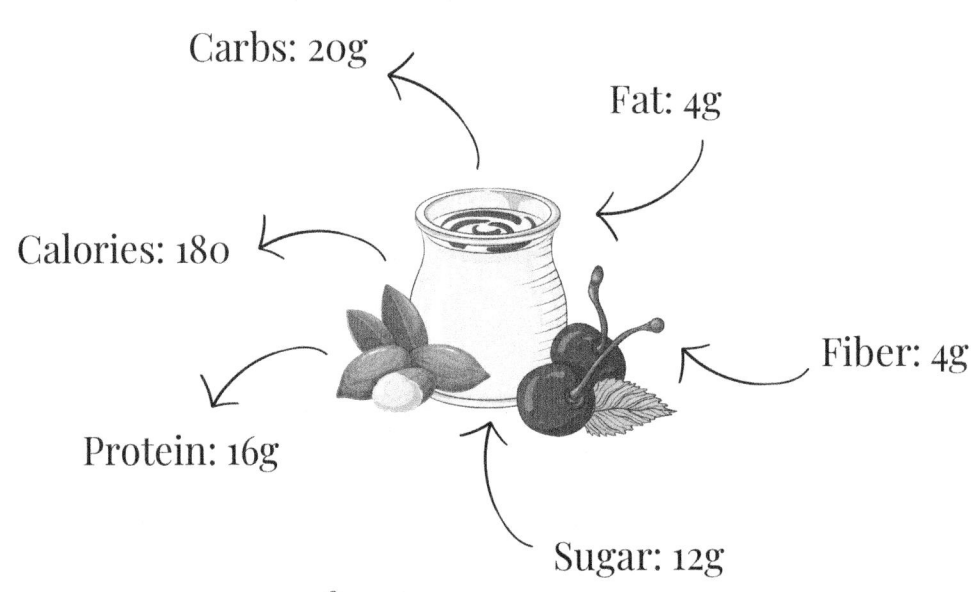

- Carbs: 20g
- Fat: 4g
- Calories: 180
- Fiber: 4g
- Protein: 16g
- Sugar: 12g

OATMEAL WITH BANANA & ALMOND BUTTER 7

This warm and hearty oatmeal breakfast is a classic for a reason. It's easy to make, filling, and provides a balanced mix of carbohydrates, protein, and healthy fats to keep you fueled all morning.

Prep: 5 mins | Cooking: 10 mins | Serve: 01

INGREDIENTS

- 1/2 cup old-fashioned rolled oats: 4 SmartPoints
- 1 cup water or milk (almond milk or skim milk works great): 0 SmartPoints for water, 1 SmartPoint for unsweetened almond milk, or 2 SmartPoints for skim milk
- 1/2 banana, sliced: 0 SmartPoints
- 1 tablespoon almond butter: 3 SmartPoints

INSTRUCTIONS

1. In a medium saucepan, bring the water or milk to a boil.
2. Add the rolled oats and reduce heat to a simmer. Cook for about 5 minutes, stirring occasionally, until the oats are thick and creamy.
3. Top the oatmeal with sliced banana and almond butter.
4. Serve and enjoy!

NUTRITIONS

Approximate, based on using 1/2 cup of old-fashioned rolled oats, 1 cup of unsweetened almond milk, 1/2 banana, and 1 tablespoon of almond butter

- Carbs: 45g
- Fat: 12g
- Calories: 320
- Fiber: 8g
- Protein: 10g
- Sugar: 10g

AVOCADO TOAST WITH A POACHED EGG & TOMATO 7

This hearty breakfast features creamy avocado, a perfectly poached egg, and juicy tomato slices on top of whole grain toast. It's an easy and satisfying breakfast that provides a good balance of protein, healthy fats, and complex carbohydrates.

Prep: 10 mins **Cooking:** 5-10 mins **Serve:** 01

INGREDIENTS

- 1 slice whole grain bread, toasted: 2 SmartPoints
- 1/2 avocado, mashed: 5 SmartPoints
- 1 egg, poached: 0 SmartPoints
- 1 tomato, sliced: 0 SmartPoints
- Salt and pepper, to taste: 0 SmartPoints

INSTRUCTIONS

1. Toast the bread until crispy and golden.
2. Mash the avocado with a fork and spread it onto the toast.
3. Top the avocado with the sliced tomato.
4. Poach an egg and place it on top of the tomato.
5. Sprinkle with salt and pepper, to taste.
6. Serve and enjoy!

NUTRITIONS

Approximate, based on using 1 slice of whole grain bread, 1/2 avocado, 1 poached egg, and 1 medium tomato

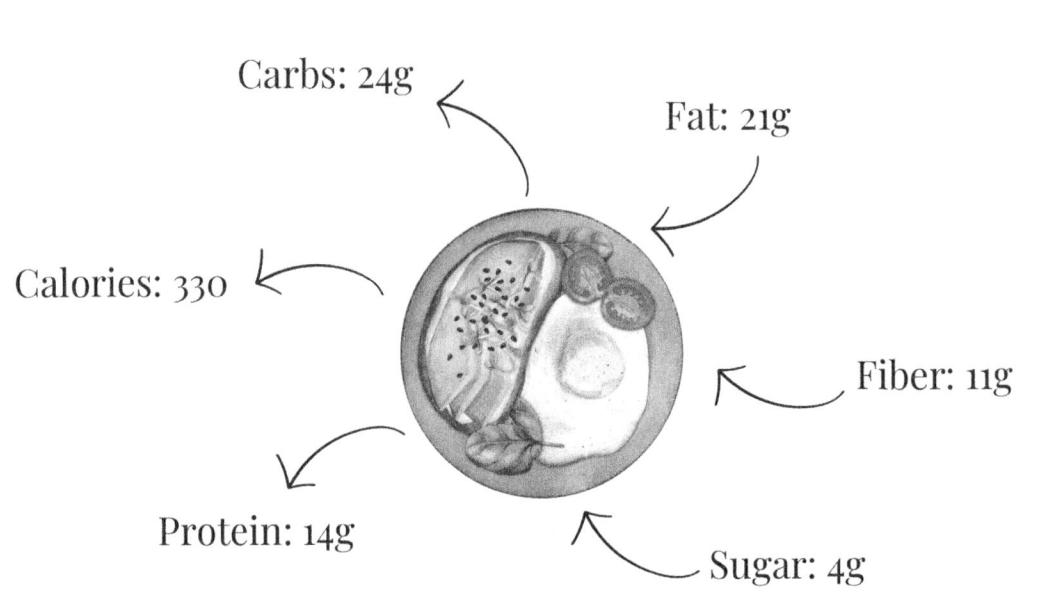

Carbs: 24g
Fat: 21g
Calories: 330
Fiber: 11g
Protein: 14g
Sugar: 4g

SMOOTHIE BOWL WITH MIXED BERRIES, BANANA, & SPINACH 3

This nutrient-packed smoothie bowl is a refreshing and delicious way to start your day. The combination of mixed berries, banana, and spinach provides a healthy dose of antioxidants, fiber, and vitamins, while the almond milk and chia seeds add protein and healthy fats.

Prep: 5-10 mins   Cooking: 0 mins   Serve: 01

— INGREDIENTS —

- 1 cup frozen mixed berries: 0 SmartPoints
- 1 banana, sliced: 0 SmartPoints
- 1 cup fresh spinach leaves: 0 SmartPoints
- 1/2 cup unsweetened almond milk: 1 SmartPoint
- 1 tablespoon chia seeds: 2 SmartPoints
- Optional toppings: sliced almonds, sliced banana, fresh berries

— INSTRUCTIONS —

1. In a blender, combine the frozen mixed berries, sliced banana, fresh spinach leaves, almond milk, and chia seeds. Blend until smooth and creamy.
2. Pour the smoothie into a bowl.
3. Top with sliced almonds, sliced banana, and fresh berries, if desired.
4. Serve and enjoy!

NUTRITIONS

- Carbs: 44g
- Fat: 3g
- Calories: 288
- Fiber: 8g
- Protein: 16g
- Sugar: 31g

VEGGIE OMELET WITH MUSHROOMS, SPINACH, & BELL PEPPERS 1

This veggie-packed omelet is a nutritious and delicious way to start your day. It's loaded with protein, fiber, and vitamins and minerals from the colorful array of vegetables.

Prep: 10 mins | Cooking: 5-10 mins | Serve: 01

— INGREDIENTS —

- 2 eggs: 0 SmartPoints
- 1/2 cup sliced mushrooms: 0 SmartPoints
- 1/2 cup fresh spinach leaves: 0 SmartPoints
- 1/4 cup chopped bell peppers: 0 SmartPoints
- Salt and pepper, to taste: 0 SmartPoints
- 1 teaspoon olive oil: 1 SmartPoint

—INSTRUCTIONS—

1. In a small bowl, whisk together the eggs with salt and pepper.
2. Heat the olive oil in a non-stick skillet over medium heat.
3. Add the sliced mushrooms, spinach leaves, and chopped bell peppers to the skillet and cook until the vegetables are soft, about 5 minutes.
4. Pour the whisked eggs over the vegetables and cook until the eggs are set, about 3-4 minutes.
5. Use a spatula to fold the omelet in half, and slide it onto a plate.
6. Serve and enjoy!

NUTRITIONS

Approximate, based on using 2 eggs, 1/2 cup sliced mushrooms, 1/2 cup fresh spinach, 1/4 cup chopped bell peppers, and 1 teaspoon olive oil

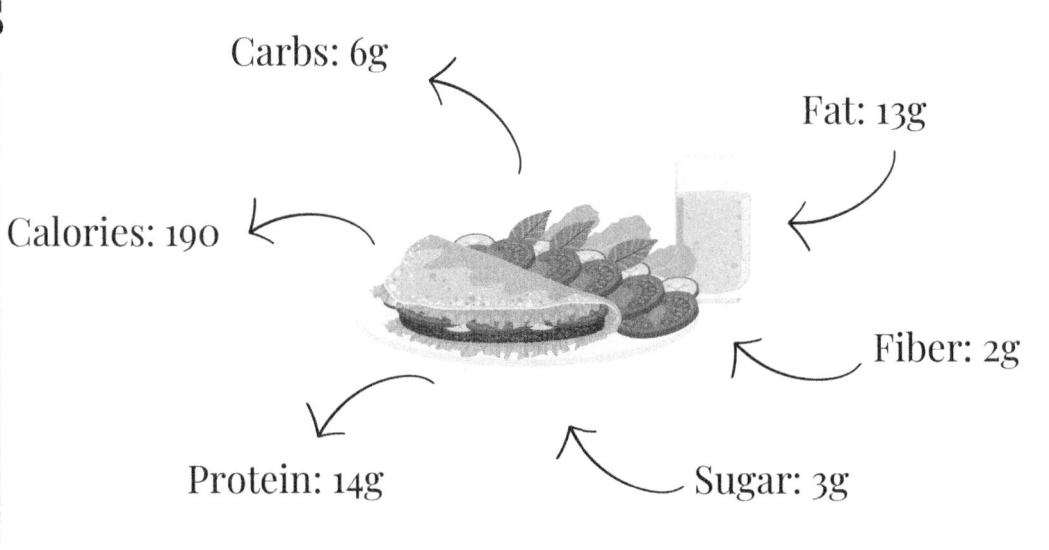

- Carbs: 6g
- Fat: 13g
- Calories: 190
- Fiber: 2g
- Protein: 14g
- Sugar: 3g

WHOLE GRAIN ENGLISH MUFFIN WITH TURKEY BACON, TOMATO, & SCRAMBLED EGG WHITES 5

This protein-packed breakfast sandwich features a whole grain English muffin, crispy turkey bacon, juicy tomato slices, and fluffy scrambled egg whites. It's a satisfying and easy breakfast that provides a good balance of complex carbohydrates, lean protein, and healthy fats.

Prep: 10-14 mins   Cooking: 7-9 mins   Serve: 01

INGREDIENTS

- 1 whole grain English muffin: 4 SmartPoints
- 2 slices turkey bacon: 1 SmartPoint
- 2 egg whites: 0 SmartPoints
- 1/2 medium tomato, sliced: 0 SmartPoints
- Salt and pepper, to taste: 0 SmartPoints

INSTRUCTIONS

1. Toast the whole grain English muffin until crispy and golden.
2. Cook the turkey bacon in a non-stick skillet over medium heat until crispy, about 3-4 minutes per side.
3. Remove the turkey bacon from the skillet and set aside.
4. In a small bowl, whisk the egg whites with salt and pepper.
5. Add the whisked egg whites to the skillet and cook until scrambled, about 2-3 minutes.
6. Assemble the sandwich by placing the turkey bacon, scrambled egg whites, and tomato slices on top of the toasted English muffin.
7. Serve and enjoy!

NUTRITIONS

Approximate, based on using 1 whole grain English muffin, 2 slices turkey bacon, 2 egg whites, and 1/2 medium tomato

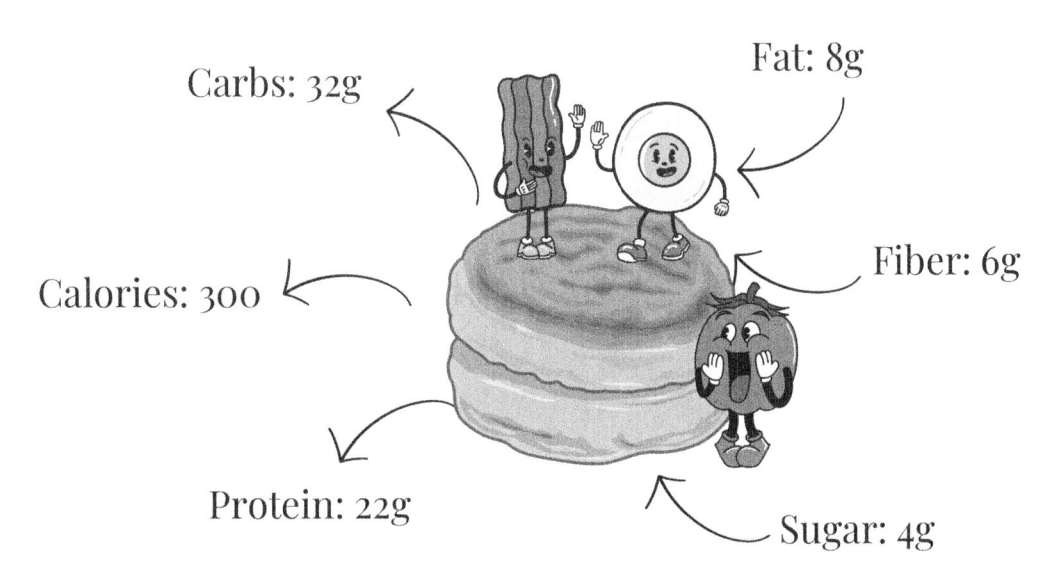

- Carbs: 32g
- Fat: 8g
- Fiber: 6g
- Calories: 300
- Protein: 22g
- Sugar: 4g

COTTAGE CHEESE WITH SLICED PEACHES & A DRIZZLE OF HONEY

3

This simple and delicious breakfast features creamy cottage cheese, juicy sliced peaches, and a drizzle of honey for sweetness. It's a satisfying breakfast that provides a good balance of protein, complex carbohydrates, and healthy fats.

Prep: 2-3 mins | Cooking: 0 min | Serve: 01

— INGREDIENTS —

- 1/2 cup low-fat cottage cheese: 2 SmartPoints
- 1 medium peach, sliced: 0 SmartPoints
- 1 teaspoon honey: 1 SmartPoint

— INSTRUCTIONS —

1. In a bowl, spoon the low-fat cottage cheese.
2. Top the cottage cheese with sliced peaches.
3. Drizzle the honey over the peaches.
4. Serve and enjoy!

NUTRITIONS

Approximate, based on using 1/2 cup low-fat cottage cheese, 1 medium peach, and 1 teaspoon honey

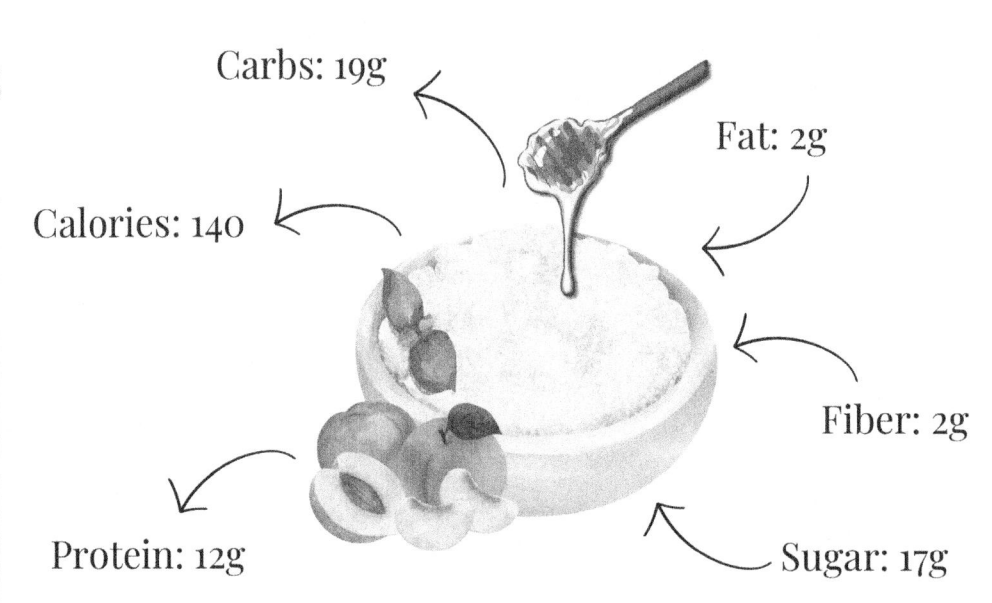

Carbs: 19g
Fat: 2g
Calories: 140
Fiber: 2g
Sugar: 17g
Protein: 12g

HIGH-FIBER CEREAL WIT ALMOND MILK & SLICED BANANA [3]

This simple and quick breakfast features high-fiber cereal, unsweetened almond milk, and sliced banana. It's a satisfying breakfast that provides a good balance of complex carbohydrates, fiber, and healthy fats.

Prep: 1-2 mins | Cooking: 0 min | Serve: 01

—— INGREDIENTS ——

- 1/2 cup low-fat cottage cheese: 2 SmartPoints
- 1 medium peach, sliced: 0 SmartPoints
- 1 teaspoon honey: 1 SmartPoint

—— INSTRUCTIONS ——

1. In a bowl, pour the high-fiber cereal.
2. Pour the unsweetened almond milk over the cereal.
3. Top the cereal with sliced banana.
4. Serve and enjoy!

NUTRITIONS

Approximate, based on using 1 cup high-fiber cereal, 1/2 cup unsweetened almond milk, and 1/2 medium banana

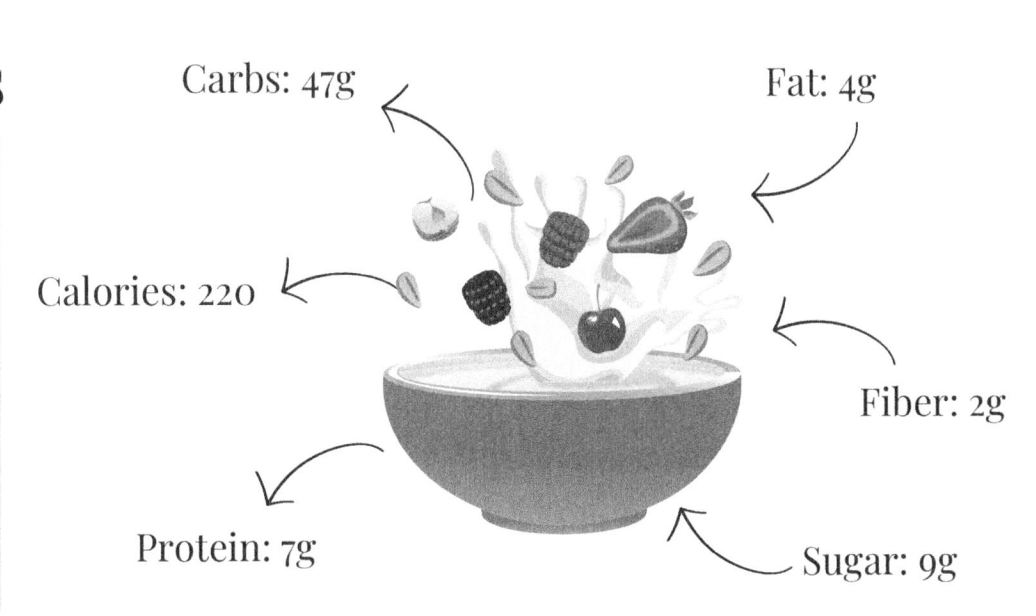

- Carbs: 47g
- Fat: 4g
- Calories: 220
- Fiber: 2g
- Protein: 7g
- Sugar: 9g

SWEET POTATO & BLACK BEAN BURRITO WITH SALSA 6

This delicious and filling breakfast burrito features sweet potatoes, black beans, eggs, and salsa wrapped in a whole wheat tortilla. It's a satisfying and nutritious breakfast that provides a good balance of complex carbohydrates, fiber, and protein.

Prep: 27-34 mins | Cooking: 3-5 min | Serve: 01

INGREDIENTS

- 1 medium sweet potato, peeled and diced: 3 SmartPoints
- 1/2 tablespoon olive oil: 1 SmartPoint
- 1/4 teaspoon cumin: 0 SmartPoints
- 1/4 teaspoon chili powder: 0 SmartPoints
- 1/4 teaspoon paprika: 0 SmartPoints
- 1/4 teaspoon salt: 0 SmartPoints
- 1/2 cup canned black beans, rinsed and drained: 0 SmartPoints
- 2 eggs, scrambled: 0 SmartPoints
- 1 whole wheat tortilla: 2 SmartPoints
- 2 tablespoons salsa: 0 SmartPoints

INSTRUCTIONS

1. Preheat the oven to 400°F.
2. In a bowl, toss the diced sweet potatoes with olive oil, cumin, chili powder, paprika, and salt.
3. Spread the sweet potatoes on a baking sheet and bake for 20-25 minutes, or until tender and golden brown.
4. In a non-stick skillet over medium heat, add the black beans and cook for 2-3 minutes until heated through.
5. Add the scrambled eggs to the skillet and cook until fully cooked and scrambled, about 2-3 minutes.
6. To assemble the burrito, lay the tortilla flat and add the sweet potatoes, black beans, and scrambled eggs down the center of the tortilla.
7. Top with salsa, and wrap the tortilla around the filling.
8. Serve and enjoy!

NUTRITIONS

Approximate, based on using 1 medium sweet potato, 1/2 cup black beans, 2 eggs, 1 whole wheat tortilla, and 2 tablespoons salsa

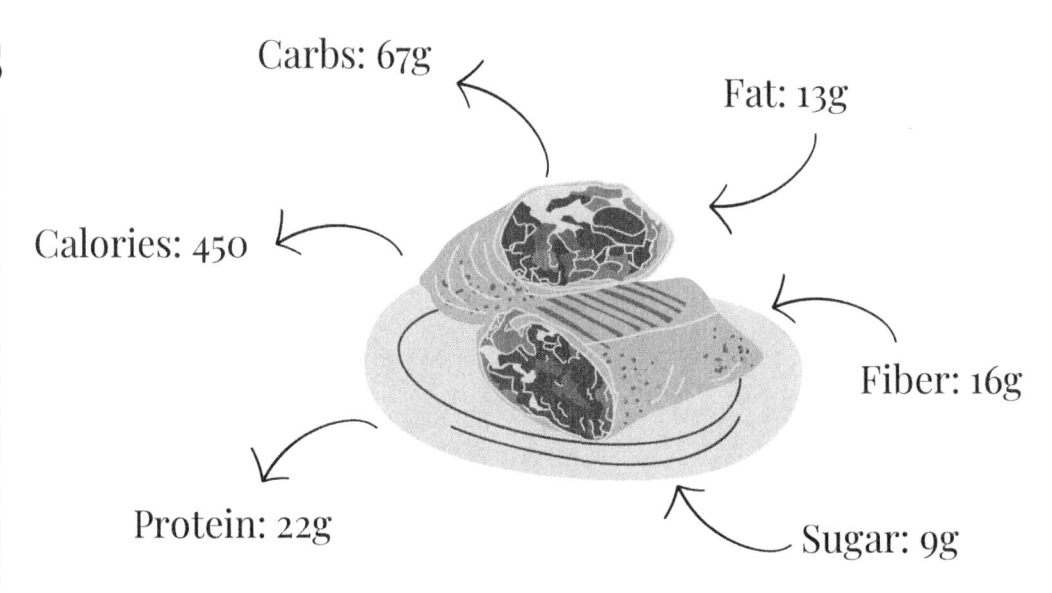

- Carbs: 67g
- Fat: 13g
- Calories: 450
- Fiber: 16g
- Protein: 22g
- Sugar: 9g

BAKED EGG CUPS WITH SPINACH AND FETA CHEESE 4

These individual baked egg cups are packed with protein and flavor, thanks to the spinach and feta cheese. They're a great make-ahead breakfast that can be reheated on busy mornings.

Prep: 1-2 mins | Cooking: 0 min | Serve: 01

INGREDIENTS

- Cooking spray: 0 SmartPoints
- 4 large eggs: 0 SmartPoints
- 1/4 cup milk: 1 SmartPoint
- 1/4 teaspoon salt: 0 SmartPoints
- 1/4 teaspoon black pepper: 0 SmartPoints
- 1/4 cup crumbled feta cheese: 3 SmartPoints
- 1/4 cup chopped spinach: 0 SmartPoints

INSTRUCTIONS

1. Preheat the oven to 375°F.
2. Spray a muffin tin with cooking spray.
3. In a bowl, whisk the eggs, milk, salt, and black pepper.
4. Stir in the feta cheese and chopped spinach.
5. Pour the egg mixture into the muffin tin, filling each cup about 3/4 full.
6. Bake for 20-25 minutes, or until the egg cups are set and golden brown.
7. Let cool for a few minutes before removing from the muffin tin.
8. Serve and enjoy!

NUTRITIONS

Approximate, based on using 4 large eggs, 1/4 cup milk, 1/4 cup crumbled feta cheese, and 1/4 cup chopped spinach

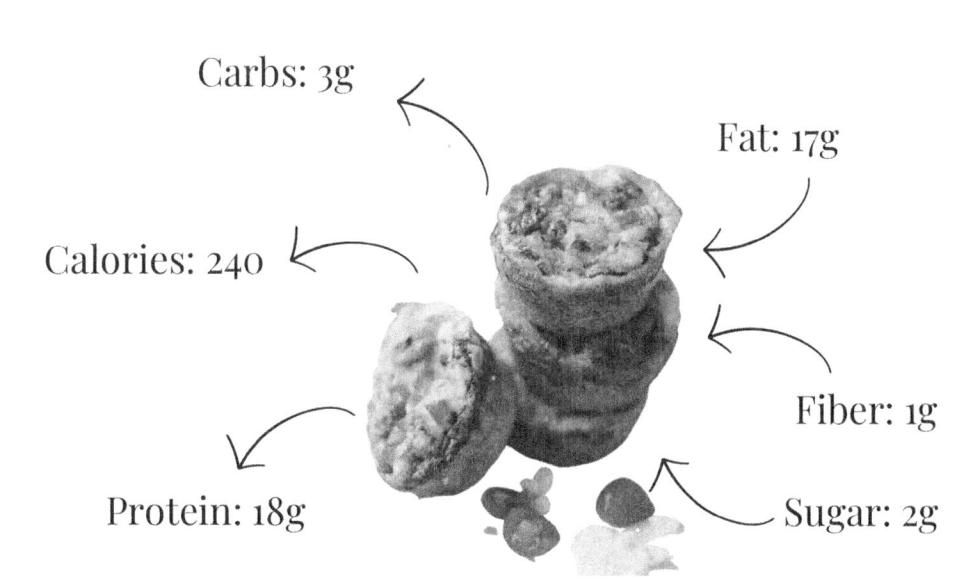

- Carbs: 3g
- Fat: 17g
- Calories: 240
- Fiber: 1g
- Protein: 18g
- Sugar: 2g

TOFU SCRAMBLE WITH VEGGIES & WHOLE WHEAT TOAST 3

This plant-based breakfast scramble is a great alternative to traditional scrambled eggs. It's made with tofu, veggies, and spices, and served with whole wheat toast. This breakfast is high in protein, fiber, and complex carbohydrates, and provides a good balance of vitamins and minerals.

Prep: 17-25 mins

Cooking: 12-15 mins

Serve: 01

INGREDIENTS

- 1/2 block of firm tofu: 0 SmartPoints
- 1/4 cup diced onion: 0 SmartPoints
- 1/4 cup diced bell pepper: 0 SmartPoints
- 1/4 cup sliced mushrooms: 0 SmartPoints
- 1 teaspoon olive oil: 1 SmartPoint
- 1/2 teaspoon turmeric: 0 SmartPoints
- 1/2 teaspoon paprika: 0 SmartPoints
- Salt and pepper to taste: 0 SmartPoints
- 1 slice of whole wheat toast: 2 SmartPoints

INSTRUCTIONS

1. In a non-stick skillet over medium heat, add the olive oil, onion, bell pepper, and mushrooms, and cook for 2-3 minutes until tender.
2. Crumble the tofu into the skillet and stir well to combine with the veggies.
3. Add the turmeric, paprika, salt, and pepper, and stir well to combine.
4. Cook for 5-7 minutes, stirring occasionally, until the tofu is heated through and slightly browned.
5. Toast the whole wheat bread.
6. Serve the tofu scramble with the toast and enjoy!

NUTRITIONS

Approximate, based on using 1/2 block of firm tofu, 1 slice of whole wheat toast, 1/4 cup diced onion, 1/4 cup diced bell pepper, and 1/4 cup sliced mushrooms

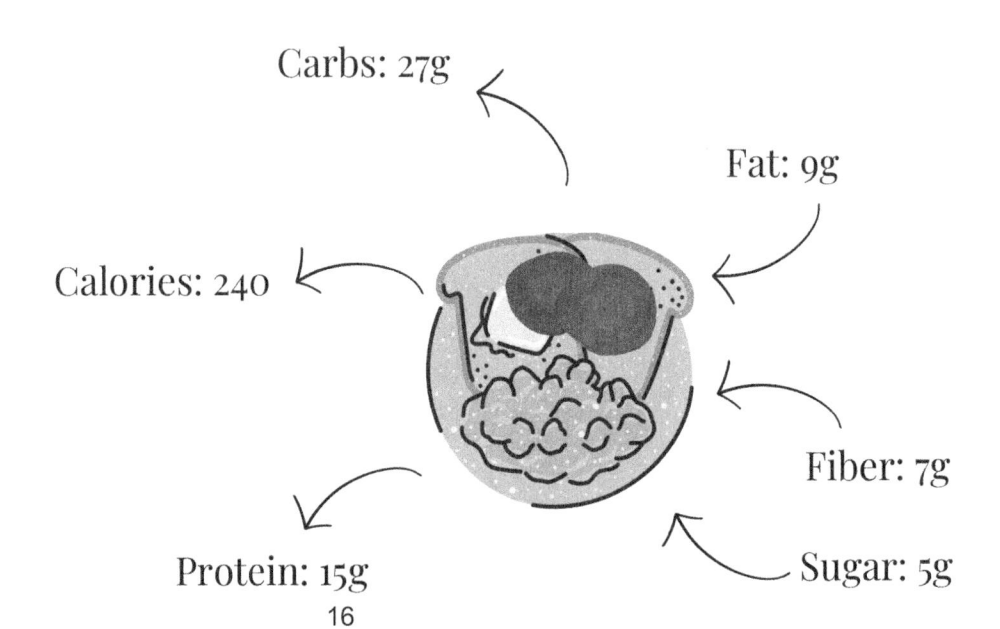

Carbs: 27g
Fat: 9g
Calories: 240
Fiber: 7g
Sugar: 5g
Protein: 15g

PEANUT BUTTER & BANANA WRAP WITH A SIDE OF FRUIT `3`

This quick and easy breakfast wrap is perfect for busy mornings. It's made with peanut butter, banana, a whole wheat tortilla, and served with a side of fruit. This breakfast is high in protein, fiber, and healthy fats, providing a good balance of vitamins & minerals.

Prep: 3-5 mins **Cooking:** 0.5 - 1 min **Serve:** 01

— INGREDIENTS —

- 1 whole wheat tortilla: 2 SmartPoints
- 2 tablespoons peanut butter: 6 SmartPoints
- 1 banana, sliced: 0 SmartPoints
- 1/2 cup mixed fruit: 0 SmartPoints

— INSTRUCTIONS —

1. Lay the whole wheat tortilla flat and spread the peanut butter evenly over the surface.
2. Add the sliced banana down the center of the tortilla.
3. Roll the tortilla up tightly, tucking in the ends as you go.
4. Slice the wrap in half and serve with a side of mixed fruit.

NUTRITIONS

Approximate, based on using 1 whole wheat tortilla, 2 tablespoons peanut butter, 1 banana, and 1/2 cup mixed fruit

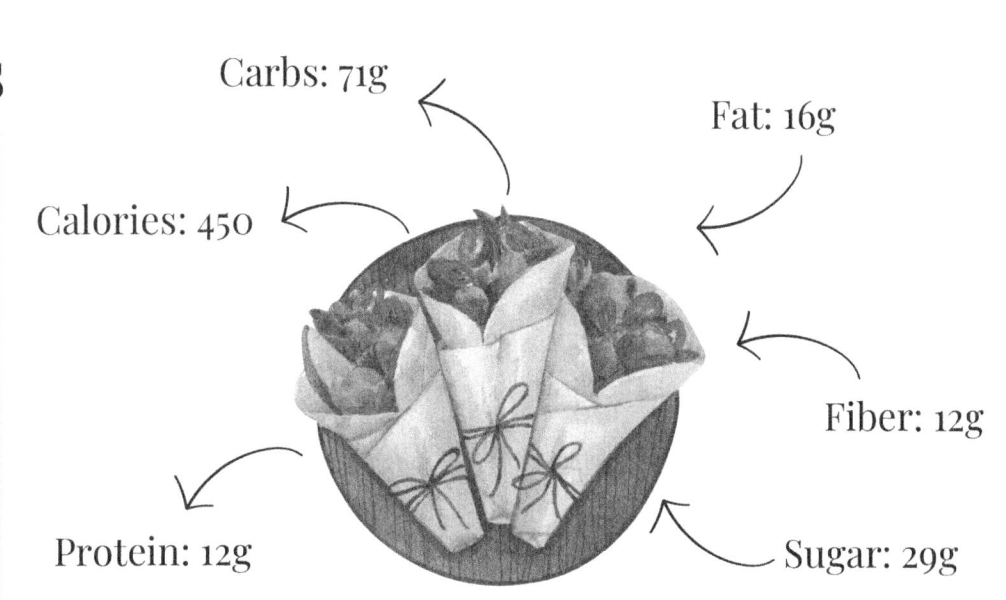

- Carbs: 71g
- Fat: 16g
- Calories: 450
- Fiber: 12g
- Protein: 12g
- Sugar: 29g

BROILED GRAPEFRUIT WITH A SPRINKLE OF BROWN SUGAR 3

This broiled grapefruit is a simple and healthy way to add some sweetness to your breakfast. Grapefruit is a good source of vitamin C, fiber, and antioxidants, and the brown sugar adds a touch of caramelized flavor.

Prep: 2-4 mins   Cooking: 3 - 5 mins   Serve: 01

—— INGREDIENTS —— | —— INSTRUCTIONS ——

- 1 large grapefruit, halved: 0 SmartPoints
- 1 tablespoon brown sugar: 3 SmartPoints

1. Preheat the broiler to high.
2. Place the grapefruit halves, cut side up, on a baking sheet.
3. Sprinkle each half with brown sugar.
4. Place the baking sheet under the broiler and broil for 3-5 minutes, or until the sugar is bubbly and the grapefruit is lightly browned.
5. Remove from the oven and let cool for a few minutes before serving.

NUTRITIONS

Approximate, based on using 1 large grapefruit and 1 tablespoon of brown sugar

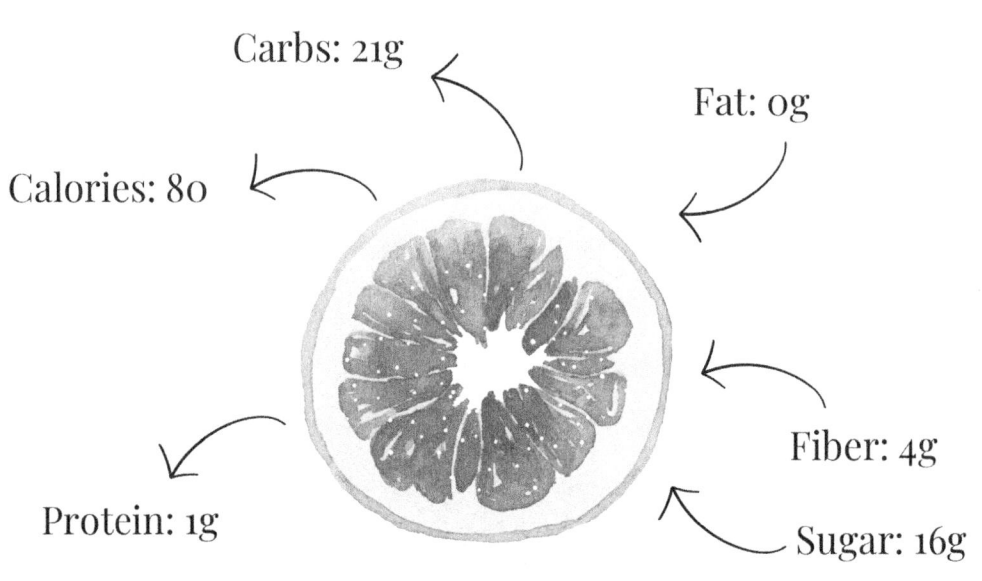

Carbs: 21g
Fat: 0g
Calories: 80
Fiber: 4g
Sugar: 16g
Protein: 1g

LOW-FAT PLAIN YOGURT WITH HONEY, WALNUTS, SLICED PEAR 5

This low-fat yogurt breakfast is a tasty and healthy way to start your day. It's full of protein, fiber, and healthy fats, and the sweet and nutty toppings make it feel like a treat.

Prep: 2-4 mins | Cooking: 0 min | Serve: 01

INGREDIENTS

- 1/2 cup low-fat plain yogurt: 2 SmartPoints
- 1/2 pear, sliced: 0 SmartPoints
- 1 tablespoon chopped walnuts: 2 SmartPoints
- 1 teaspoon honey: 1 SmartPoint

INSTRUCTIONS

1. Spoon the low-fat plain yogurt into a breakfast bowl.
2. Top with the sliced pear and chopped walnuts.
3. Drizzle with honey.
4. Serve and enjoy!

NUTRITIONS

Approximate, based on using 1/2 cup of low-fat plain yogurt, 1/2 pear, 1 tablespoon of chopped walnuts, and 1 teaspoon of honey

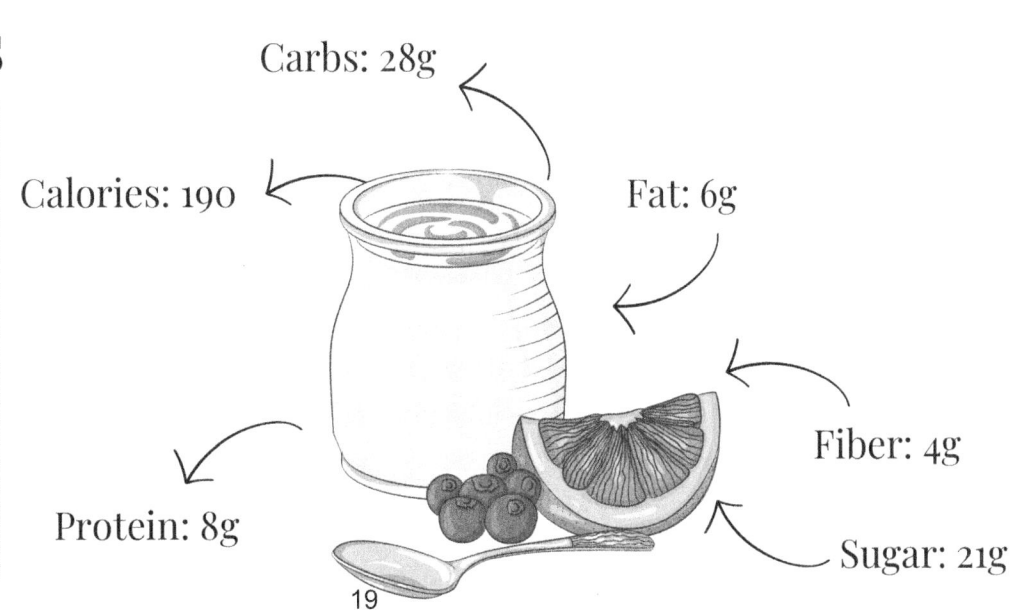

- Carbs: 28g
- Calories: 190
- Fat: 6g
- Fiber: 4g
- Sugar: 21g
- Protein: 8g

WHOLE WHEAT TOAST WITH AVOCADO, TOMATO, & A POACHED EGG 7

This recipe is the perfect way to start your day. Whole wheat toast is topped with creamy avocado, fresh tomato, a perfectly poached egg for a satisfying and protein-packed meal.

Prep: 7-10 mins | Cooking: 4-5 min | Serve: 01

—— INGREDIENTS ——

- 1 slice of whole wheat bread: 2 SmartPoints
- 1/2 avocado, mashed: 5 SmartPoints
- 1/2 tomato, sliced: 0 SmartPoints
- 1 egg, poached: 0 SmartPoints

—— INSTRUCTIONS ——

1. Toast the whole wheat bread to your desired level of crispiness.
2. Spread the mashed avocado on top of the toast.
3. Place the sliced tomato on top of the avocado.
4. Poach the egg to your liking and place it on top of the tomato.
5. Season with salt and pepper to taste.
6. Serve and enjoy!

NUTRITIONS

Approximate, based on using 1 slice of whole wheat bread, 1/2 avocado, 1/2 tomato, and 1 poached egg

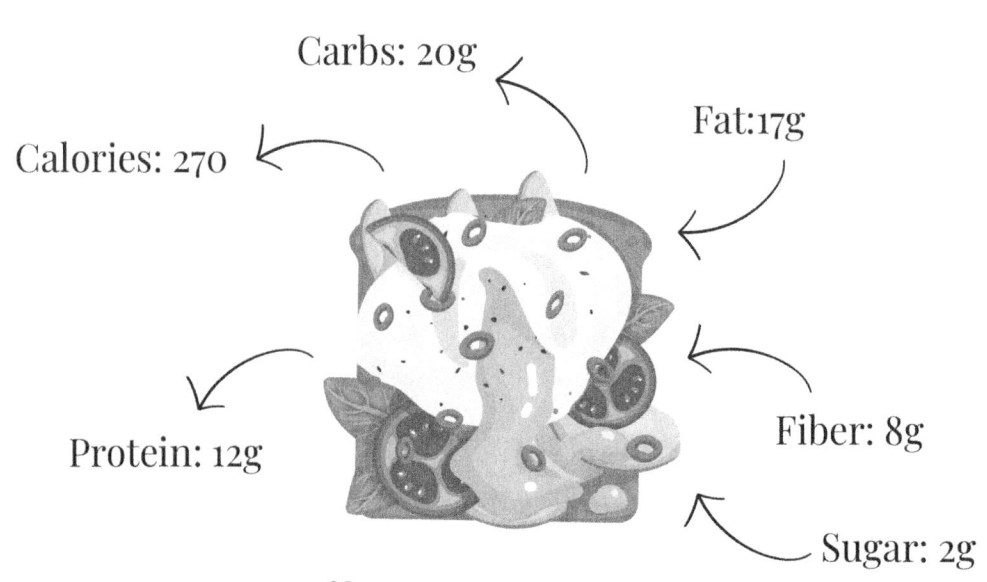

- Carbs: 20g
- Fat: 17g
- Calories: 270
- Fiber: 8g
- Protein: 12g
- Sugar: 2g

FRUIT & NUT GRANOLA WITH ALMOND MILK & MIXED BERRIES 🔲8

This recipe is the perfect way to start your day. Whole wheat toast is topped with creamy avocado, fresh tomato, a perfectly poached egg for a satisfying and protein-packed meal.

Prep: 7-10 mins | Cooking: 4-5 min | Serve: 01

— INGREDIENTS —

- 1 slice of whole wheat bread: 2 SmartPoints
- 1/2 avocado, mashed: 6 SmartPoints
- 1/2 tomato, sliced: 0 SmartPoints
- 1 poached egg: 0 SmartPoints
- Salt and pepper to taste: 0 SmartPoints

— INSTRUCTIONS —

1. Toast the whole wheat bread to your desired level of crispiness.
2. Spread the mashed avocado on top of the toast.
3. Place the sliced tomato on top of the avocado.
4. Poach the egg to your liking and place it on top of the tomato.
5. Season with salt and pepper to taste.
6. Serve and enjoy!

NUTRITIONS

Approximate, based on using 1 slice of whole wheat bread, 1/2 avocado, 1/2 tomato, and 1 poached egg

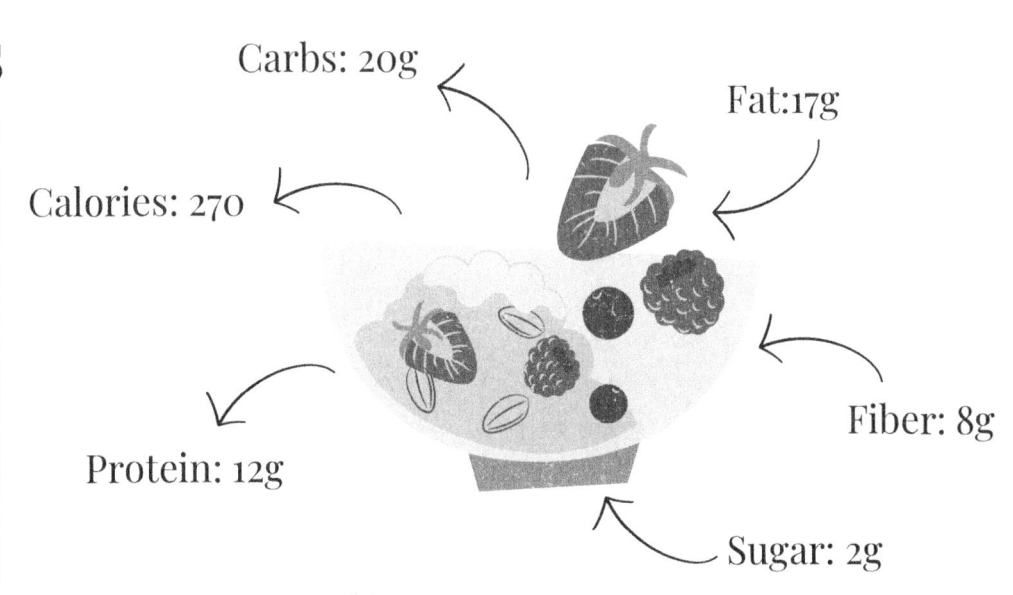

- Carbs: 20g
- Fat: 17g
- Calories: 270
- Fiber: 8g
- Protein: 12g
- Sugar: 2g

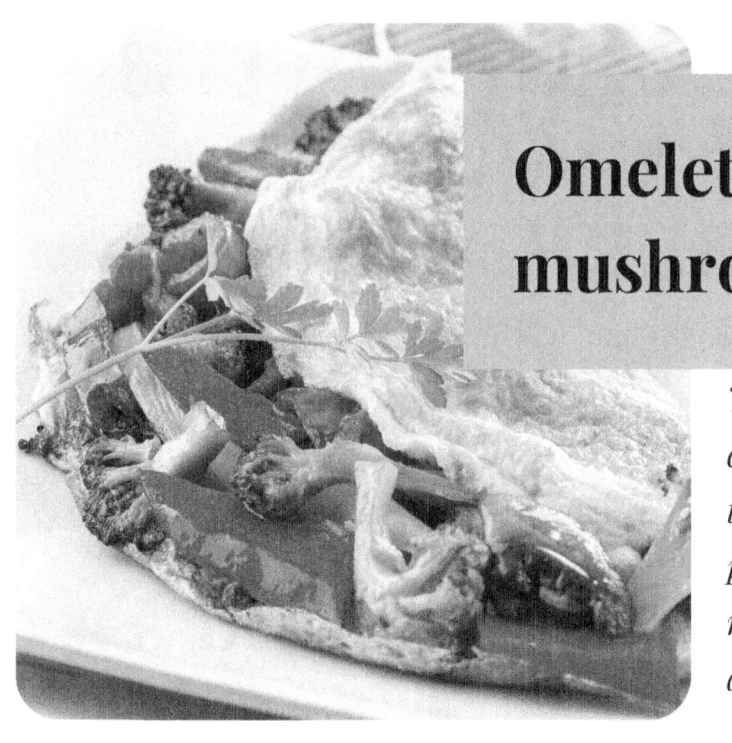

Omelet with spinach, mushrooms, & turkey bacon

This omelet recipe is high in protein and low in calories, making it a great breakfast option for those following Dr. Nowzaradan's weight loss program. The combination of spinach, mushrooms, and turkey bacon makes for a delicious and filling meal.

Serving(s): 01 **Preparing time:** 10 mins **Cooking time:** 10 mins

INGREDIENTS

- 2 large eggs: 0
- 1/4 cup sliced mushrooms: 0
- 1/4 cup fresh spinach: 0
- 1 slice of turkey bacon, chopped: 1
- 1 teaspoon olive oil: 1
- Salt and pepper to taste: 0

DIRECTIONS

1. Heat the olive oil in a non-stick pan over medium heat.
2. Add the sliced mushrooms and cook for 2-3 minutes, until they start to brown.
3. Add the chopped turkey bacon and cook for an additional 2-3 minutes.
4. Add the fresh spinach to the pan and cook until wilted.
5. Whisk the eggs in a bowl and season with salt and pepper.
6. Pour the egg mixture into the pan and cook until the edges start to set.
7. Use a spatula to lift the edges of the omelet and allow the uncooked eggs to flow underneath.
8. Once the omelet is set, fold it in half and slide it onto a plate.
9. Serve hot and enjoy!

NUTRITIONS (PER SERVING)

Calories: 213   Protein: 18g   Fat: 15g   Carbohydrates: 3g   Fiber: 1g   Sugar: 1g

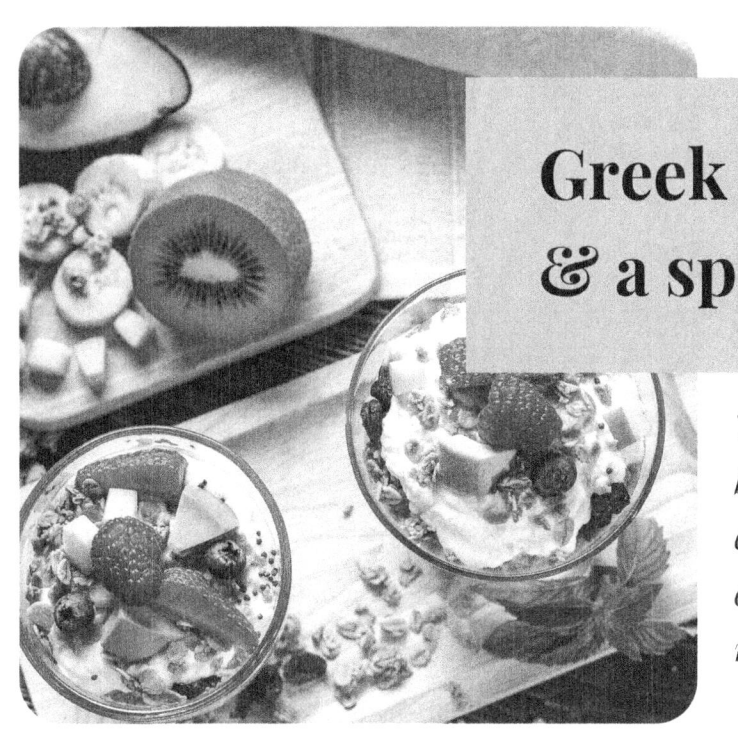

Greek yogurt with berries & a sprinkle of nuts `2`

This Greek yogurt bowl is a simple yet delicious breakfast that's high in protein and low in calories. The combination of sweet berries and crunchy nuts makes for a satisfying and nutritious meal.

Serving(s): 01 | Preparing time: 5 mins | Cooking time: 0 min

INGREDIENTS

- 1/2 cup plain Greek yogurt: 0 SmartPoints
- 1/4 cup mixed berries: 0 SmartPoints
- 1 tablespoon chopped nuts: 2 SmartPoints

DIRECTIONS

1. Place the Greek yogurt in a bowl.
2. Top with the mixed berries and chopped nuts.
3. Serve and enjoy!

NUTRITIONS (PER SERVING)

Calories: 135 | Protein: 15g | Fat: 5g | Carbohydrates: 10g | Fiber: 2g | Sugar: 7g

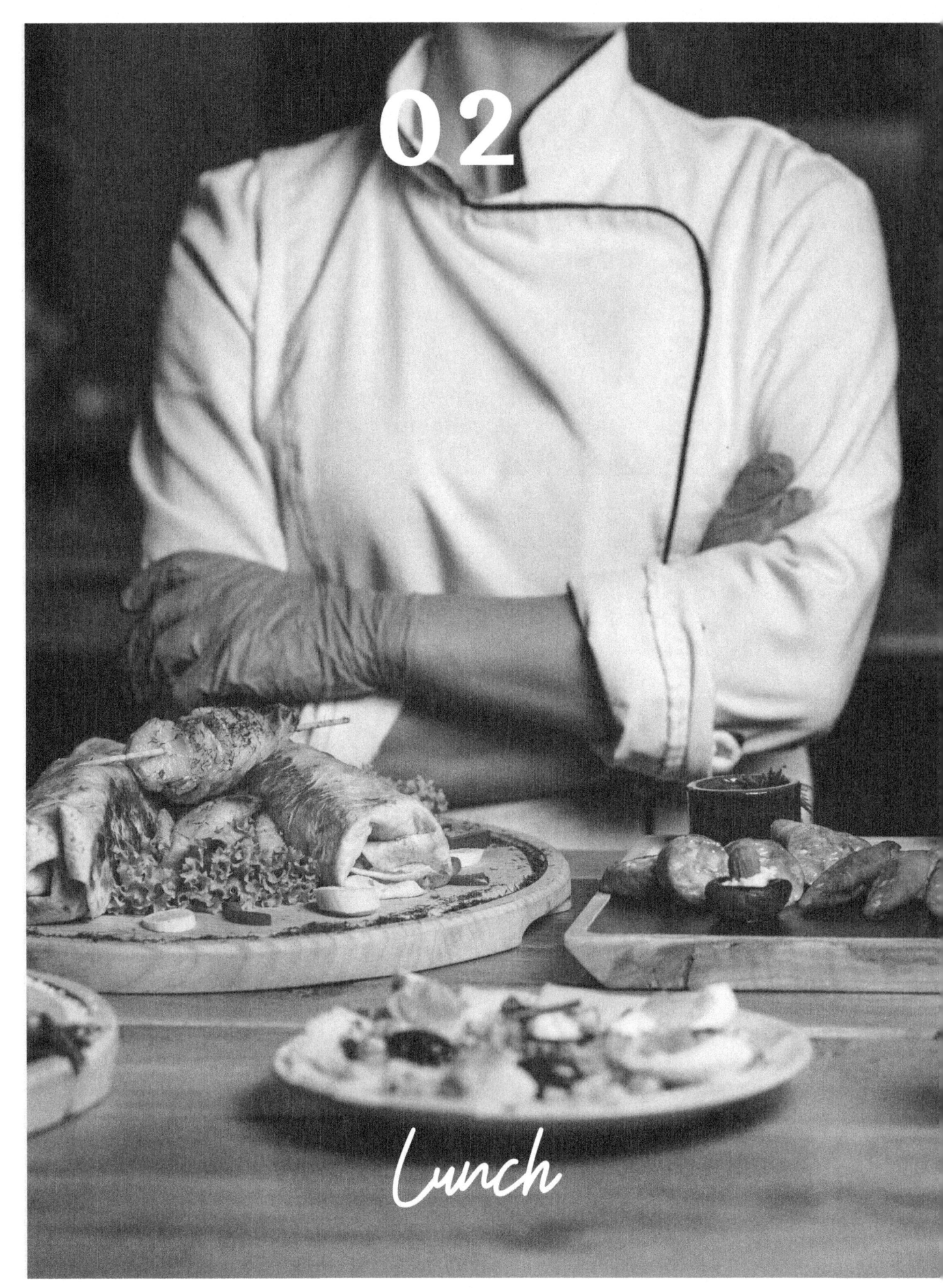

02

Lunch

Grilled chicken breast with steamed vegetables

0

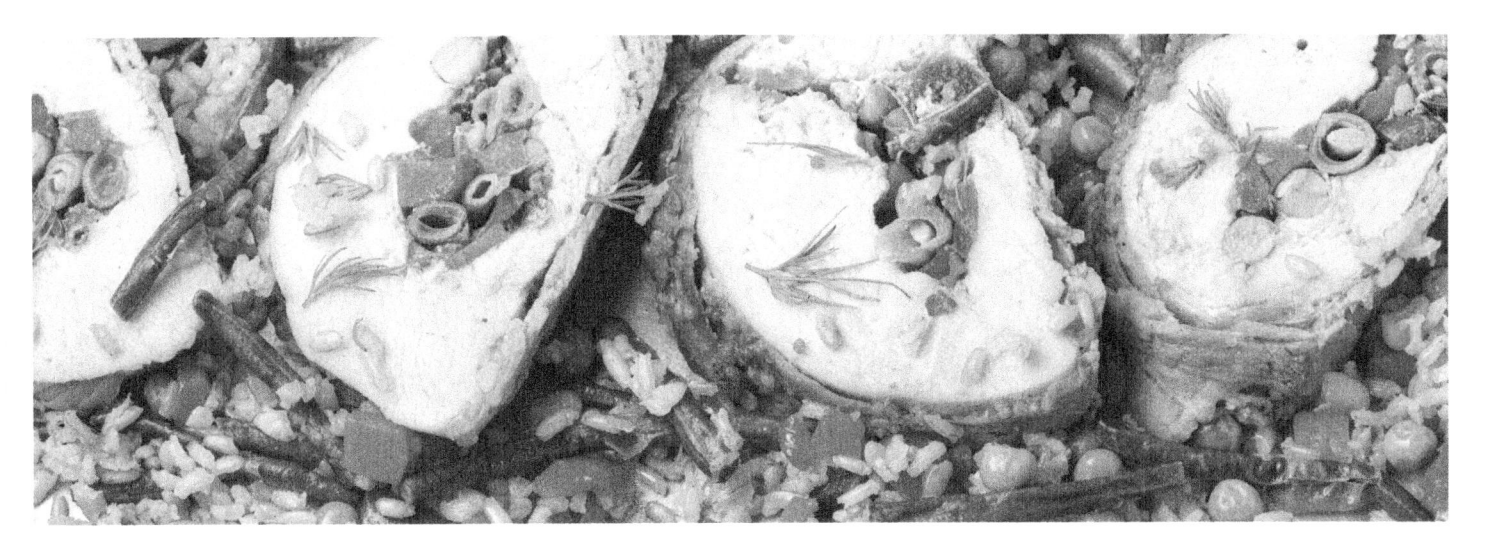

This grilled chicken breast with steamed vegetables is a simple and healthy meal that's perfect for lunch or dinner. The chicken is marinated in a flavorful blend of herbs and spices, then grilled to perfection. The vegetables are steamed until tender, and seasoned with a light sprinkling of salt and pepper.

Serving(s): 01   **Preparing time: 10 mins**   **Cooking time: 15 mins**

Ingredients

- Boneless, skinless chicken breast: 0 SmartPoints
- Garlic powder: 0 SmartPoints
- Dried oregano: 0 SmartPoints
- Dried thyme: 0 SmartPoints
- Salt and pepper: 0 SmartPoints
- Mixed vegetables: 0 SmartPoints

Directions

1. Preheat the grill to medium-high heat.
2. In a small bowl, mix together the garlic powder, dried oregano, dried thyme, salt, and pepper.
3. Season the chicken breast with the herb and spice mixture.
4. Grill the chicken breast for 6-8 minutes per side, or until cooked through.
5. While the chicken is grilling, steam the mixed vegetables until tender.
6. Serve the grilled chicken with the steamed vegetables on the side.

NUTRITIONS (PER SERVING)

Calories: 245   Protein: 32g   Fat: 8g   Carbohydrates: 10g   Fiber: 3g   Sugar: 3g

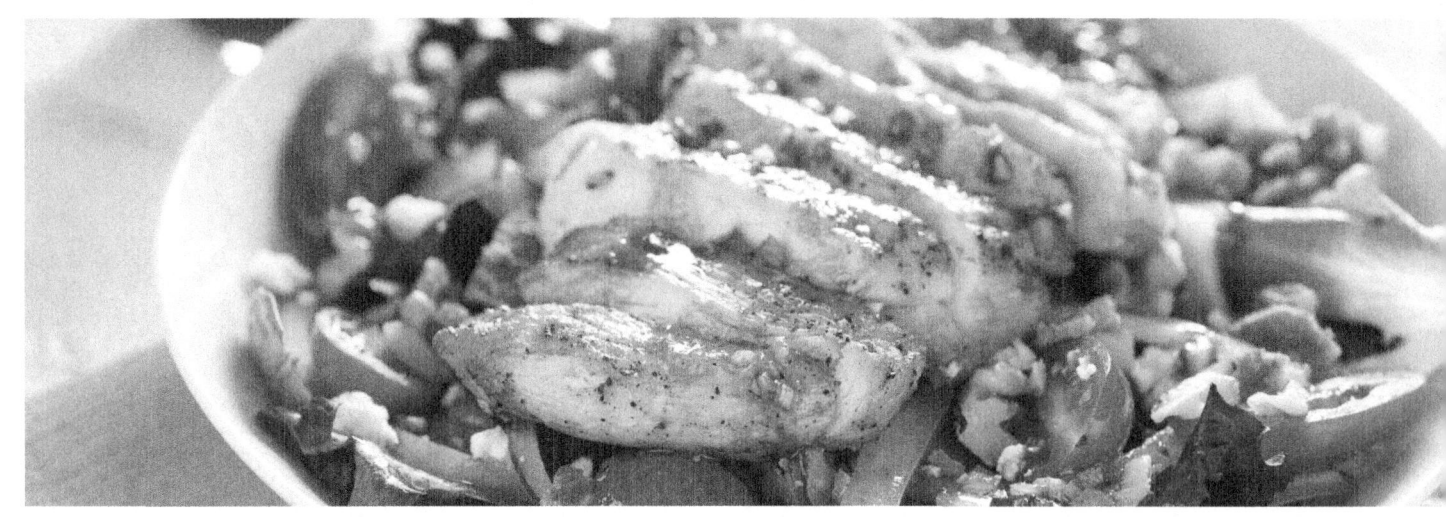

Tuna salad with mixed greens & balsamic vinaigrette dressing 5

This grilled chicken breast with steamed vegetables is a simple and healthy meal that's perfect for lunch or dinner. The chicken is marinated in a flavorful blend of herbs and spices, then grilled to perfection. The vegetables are steamed until tender, and seasoned with a light sprinkling of salt and pepper.

Serving(s): 01   **Preparing time: 10 mins**   **Cooking time: 0 min**

Ingredients

- 1 can of tuna in water, drained: 0 SmartPoints
- 2 cups mixed greens: 0 SmartPoints
- 1/4 cup chopped red onion: 0 SmartPoints
- 1/4 cup chopped celery: 0 SmartPoints
- 1/4 cup chopped cucumber: 0 SmartPoints
- 1 tablespoon olive oil: 4 SmartPoints
- 1 tablespoon balsamic vinegar: 1 SmartPoint
- Salt and pepper, to taste: 0 SmartPoints

Directions

1. In a large bowl, combine the tuna, mixed greens, red onion, celery, and cucumber.
2. In a small bowl, whisk together the olive oil, balsamic vinegar, salt, and pepper.
3. Drizzle the dressing over the tuna salad, and toss to combine.
4. Serve the salad immediately, or store it in the refrigerator for later.

NUTRITIONS (PER SERVING)

Calories: 218   Protein: 27g   Fat: 9g   Carbohydrates: 8g   Fiber: 2g

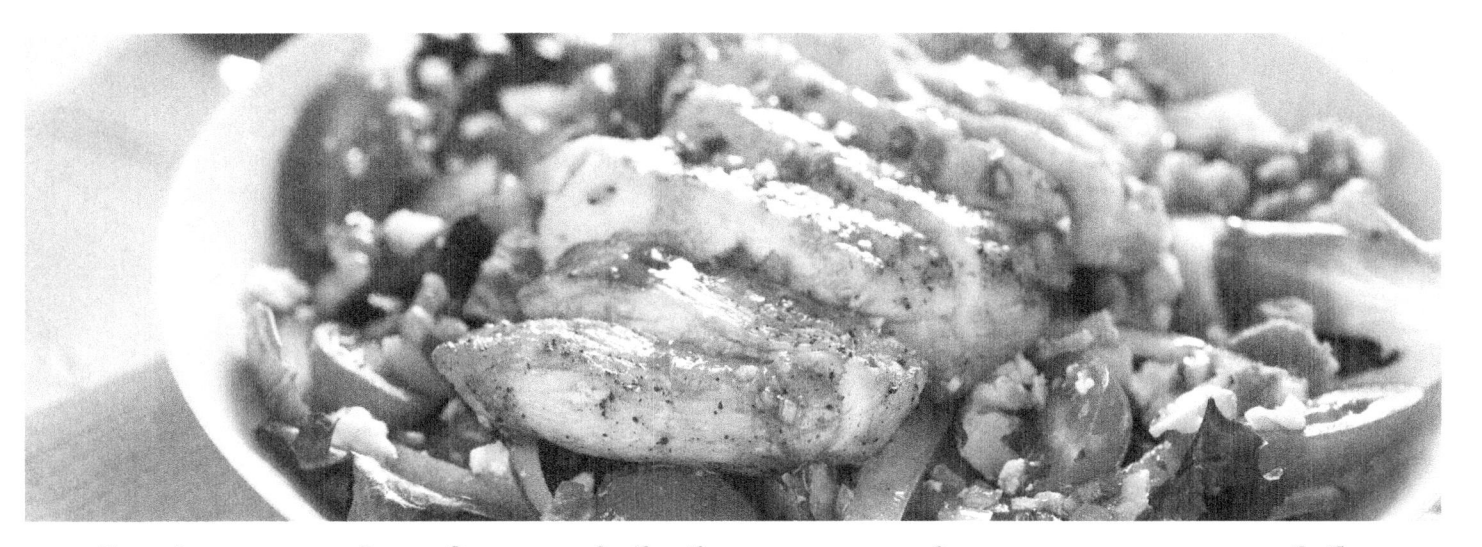

Shrimp stir-fry with brown rice & vegetables

16

This shrimp stir-fry with brown rice and vegetables is a delicious and nutritious meal that's quick and easy to prepare. The shrimp are cooked until tender and juicy, and the brown rice provides a healthy dose of fiber and carbohydrates.

Serving(s): 04   Preparing time: 10 mins   Cooking time: 20 mins

Ingredients

- 1 cup brown rice: 6 SmartPoints
- 1 pound shrimp, peeled and deveined: 0 SmartPoints
- 2 cups mixed vegetables (such as sliced bell peppers, broccoli florets, and sliced carrots): 0 SmartPoints
- 1 tablespoon vegetable oil: 4 SmartPoints
- 1 tablespoon minced garlic: 0 SmartPoints
- 1 tablespoon minced ginger: 0 SmartPoints
- 2 tablespoons soy sauce: 2 SmartPoints
- 1 tablespoon honey: 3 SmartPoints
- 1 tablespoon cornstarch: 1 SmartPoint
- Salt and pepper, to taste: 0 SmartPoints

Directions

1. Cook brown rice according to package instructions.
2. Heat the oil in a large skillet over medium-high heat.
3. Add the garlic and ginger and cook for 1-2 minutes, stirring constantly.
4. Add the vegetables and stir-fry for 2-3 minutes until they are tender-crisp.
5. Add the shrimp and cook for another 2-3 minutes until they are pink and cooked through.
6. In a small bowl, whisk together the soy sauce, honey, and cornstarch.
7. Pour the sauce over the shrimp and vegetables and stir to coat.
8. Cook for an additional 1-2 minutes until the sauce has thickened.
9. Serve the stir-fry over the brown rice.

NUTRITIONS (PER SERVING)

Calories: 389   Protein: 28g   Fat: 6g   Carbohydrates: 60g   Fiber: 6g   Sodium: 927mg

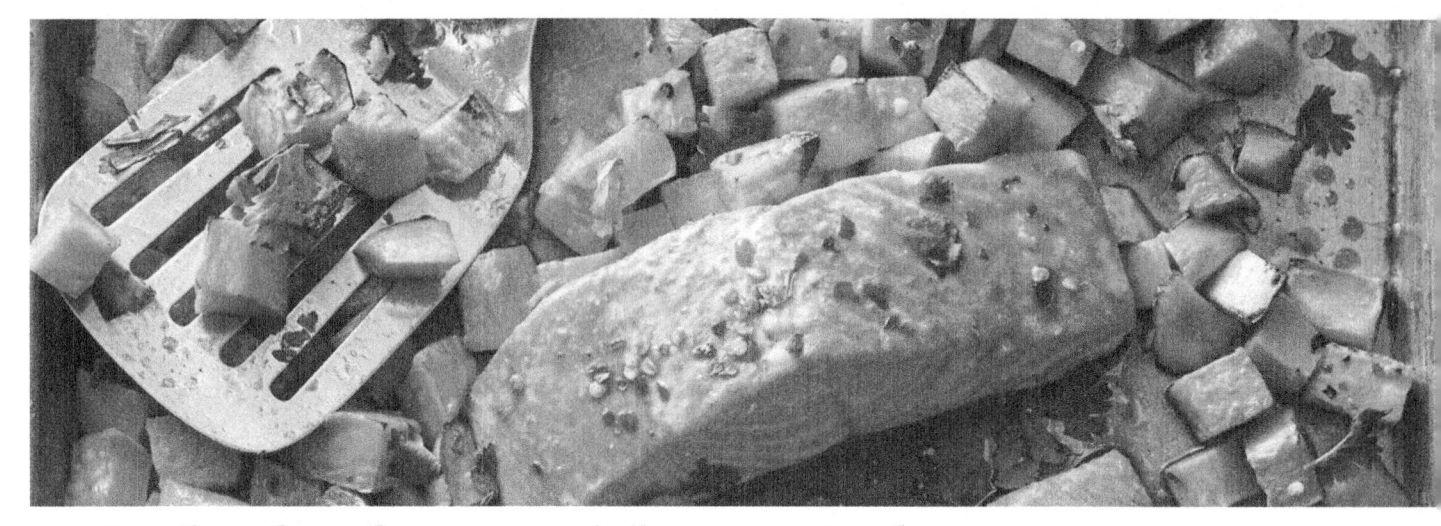

Baked salmon with roasted sweet potatoes & green beans 14

This recipe is a healthy and flavorful way to enjoy salmon, which is packed with omega-3 fatty acids. The sweet potatoes and green beans add extra fiber and nutrients to the meal.

Serving(s): 04 | Preparing time: 15 mins | Cooking time: 35 mins

Ingredients

4 salmon fillets, skin removed: 0 points

2 sweet potatoes, peeled and chopped: 6 points

2 cups green beans, trimmed: 0 points

2 tablespoons olive oil: 8 points

Salt and pepper, to taste: 0 points

Lemon wedges, for serving: 0 points

Directions

1. Preheat the oven to 400°F (200°C).
2. Line a baking sheet with parchment paper.
3. Place the sweet potatoes on one half of the baking sheet and the green beans on the other half.
4. Drizzle the vegetables with olive oil and season with salt and pepper.
5. Toss the vegetables to coat in the oil and seasoning.
6. Bake for 20-25 minutes, stirring once, until the vegetables are tender and golden brown.
7. Season the salmon fillets with salt and pepper.
8. Place the salmon on the baking sheet with the vegetables.
9. Bake for 10-12 minutes, until the salmon is cooked through and flakes easily with a fork.
10. Serve the salmon and vegetables with lemon wedges.

NUTRITIONS (PER SERVING)

Calories: 402 | Protein: 35g | Fat: 20g | Carbohydrates: 20g | Fiber: 4g | Sodium: 81mg

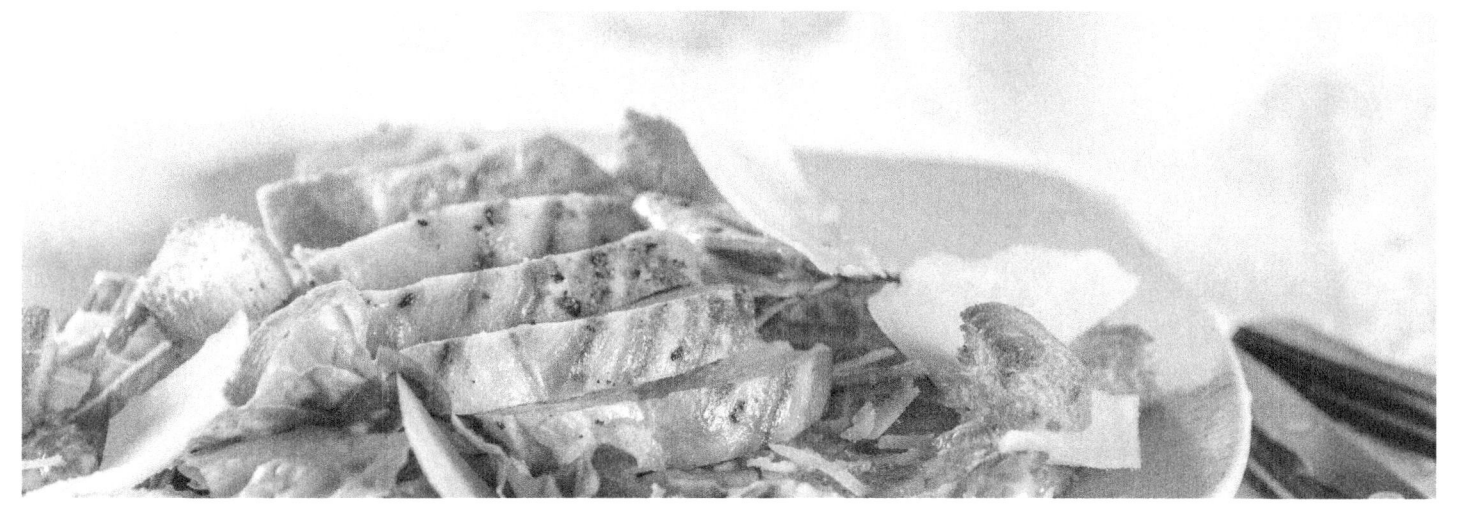

Grilled chicken Caesar salad with whole grain croutons 16

This Grilled Chicken Caesar Salad is a healthy take on the classic Caesar salad. Made with grilled chicken breast, crisp romaine lettuce, and homemade whole grain croutons, it's a satisfying and flavorful meal that's perfect for lunch.

Serving(s): 02-4　　　　Preparing time: 15 mins　　　　Cooking time: 12 mins

Ingredients

For the Salad:

Grilled chicken breasts (2) = 0 SmartPoints

Romaine lettuce, chopped = 0 SmartPoints

Grated Parmesan cheese, 1/4 cup = 4 SmartPoints

Caesar dressing, 1/4 cup = 8 SmartPoints

For the Croutons:

Whole grain bread, 2 cups cubed = 16 SmartPoints

Olive oil, 2 tablespoons = 6 SmartPoints

Garlic powder, 1/4 teaspoon = 0 SmartPoints

Salt and pepper to taste = 0 SmartPoints

Directions

1. Preheat the oven to 375°F (190°C).
2. In a bowl, mix the bread cubes, olive oil, garlic powder, salt, and pepper.
3. Spread the bread cubes evenly on a baking sheet.
4. Bake for 10-12 minutes or until golden brown.
5. In a large bowl, combine the romaine lettuce, sliced grilled chicken, grated Parmesan cheese, and Caesar dressing.
6. Add the whole grain croutons and toss to combine.
7. Serve immediately.

NUTRITIONS (PER SERVING)

Calories: 400　　Protein: 34g　　Fat: 22g　　Carbohydrates: 17g　　Fiber: 3g　　Sodium: 700mg

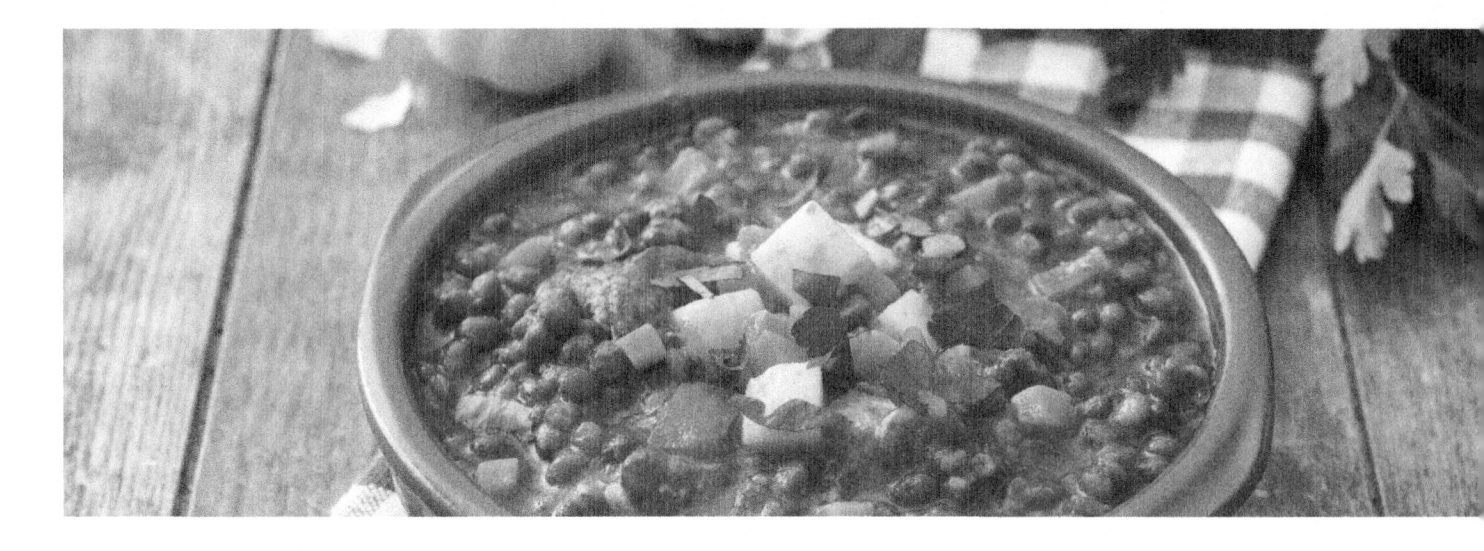

Lentil soup with mixed vegetables 10

This Lentil Soup with Mixed Vegetables is a healthy and filling lunch option. Made with protein-packed lentils, mixed vegetables, and flavorful spices, it's a comforting soup that will keep you full and satisfied throughout the day.

Serving(s): 04-6	Preparing time: 10 mins	Cooking time: 45 mins

Ingredients

- 1 cup lentils: 6 SmartPoints
- 4 cups vegetable broth: 0 SmartPoints
- 1 tablespoon olive oil: 4 SmartPoints
- 1 onion, chopped: 0 SmartPoints
- 3 cloves garlic, minced: 0 SmartPoints
- 2 carrots, chopped: 0 SmartPoints
- 2 celery stalks, chopped: 0 SmartPoints
- 1 can diced tomatoes: 0 SmartPoints
- 1 teaspoon ground cumin: 0 SmartPoints
- 1/2 teaspoon paprika: 0 SmartPoints
- Salt and pepper to taste: 0 SmartPoints

Directions

1. Rinse the lentils under running water and drain them.
2. In a large pot, heat the olive oil over medium heat.
3. Add the onion and garlic and sauté for 2-3 minutes or until softened.
4. Add the chopped carrots and celery and cook for an additional 5 minutes.
5. Add the vegetable broth, lentils, diced tomatoes, ground cumin, paprika, salt, and pepper.
6. Bring the soup to a boil, then reduce the heat to low and simmer for 30-40 minutes or until the lentils are tender.
7. Serve hot.

NUTRITIONS (PER SERVING)

Calories: 250   Protein: 16g   Fat: 3g   Carbohydrates: 43g   Fiber: 18g   Sodium: 650mg

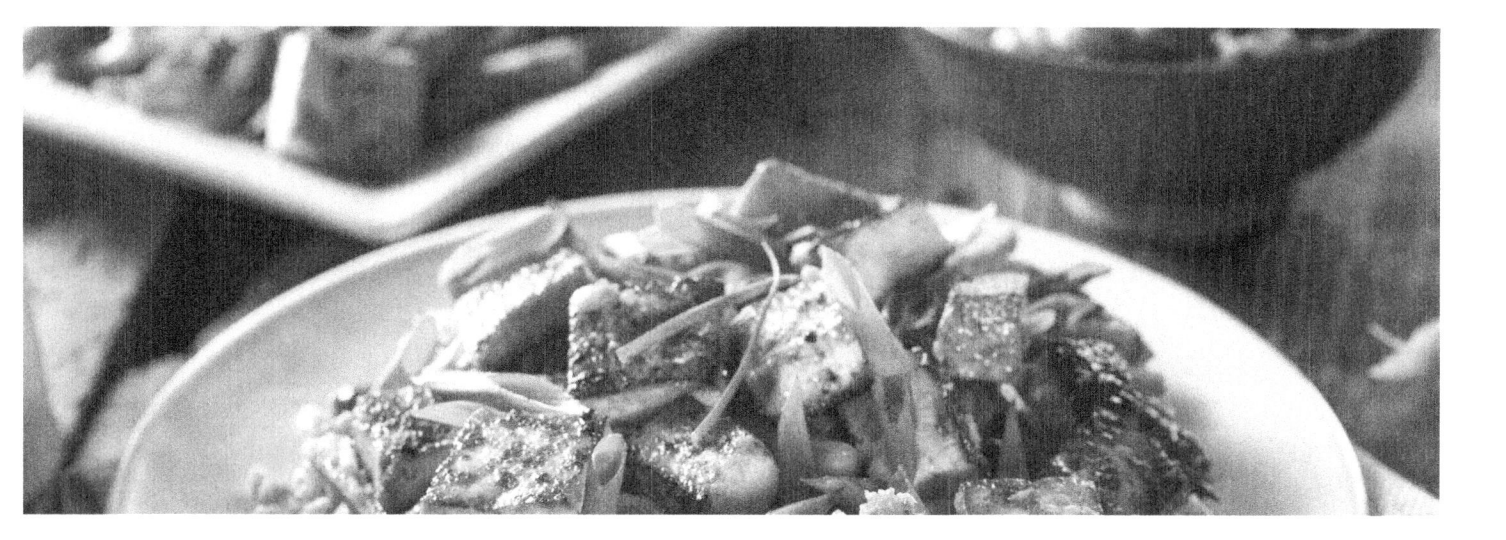

Vegetable stir-fry with tofu & brown rice [6]

This vegan recipe features a hearty and healthy black bean and vegetable chili, loaded with plant-based protein and fiber, and served with a side salad for added nutrition.

Serving(s): 04   **Preparing time: 10 mins**   **Cooking time: 20 mins**

Ingredients

- 1 tbsp olive oil: 4 SmartPoints
- 1 small onion, diced: 0 SmartPoints
- 2 cloves garlic, minced: 0 SmartPoints
- 1 bell pepper, diced: 0 SmartPoints
- 1 zucchini, diced: 0 SmartPoints
- 1 yellow squash, diced: 0 SmartPoints
- 1 can black beans, drained and rinsed: 0
- 1 can diced tomatoes: 0 SmartPoints
- 1 cup vegetable broth: 0 SmartPoints
- 1 tsp chili powder: 0 SmartPoints
- 1/2 tsp cumin: 0 SmartPoints
- Salt and pepper, to taste: 0 SmartPoints
- Fresh cilantro, chopped (optional): 0 SmartPoints
- Mixed greens or your favorite salad greens: 0 SmartPoints
- Balsamic vinaigrette dressing: 2 SmartPoints

Directions

1. Heat the olive oil in a large pot or Dutch oven over medium-high heat. Add the onion and garlic and sauté for 2-3 minutes until fragrant and translucent.
2. Add the bell pepper, zucchini, and yellow squash to the pot and sauté for an additional 3-4 minutes until slightly softened.
3. Add the black beans, diced tomatoes, vegetable broth, chili powder, cumin, salt, and pepper to the pot. Bring to a boil, then reduce the heat and let simmer for 10-15 minutes, stirring occasionally.
4. While the chili is simmering, prepare the side salad by tossing mixed greens with balsamic vinaigrette dressing.
5. Once the chili is done, ladle into bowls and sprinkle with fresh cilantro if desired. Serve alongside the side salad.

NUTRITIONS (PER SERVING)

Calories: 220   Protein: 9g   Fat: 5g   Carbohydrates: 43g   Fiber: 11g   Sugar: 7g

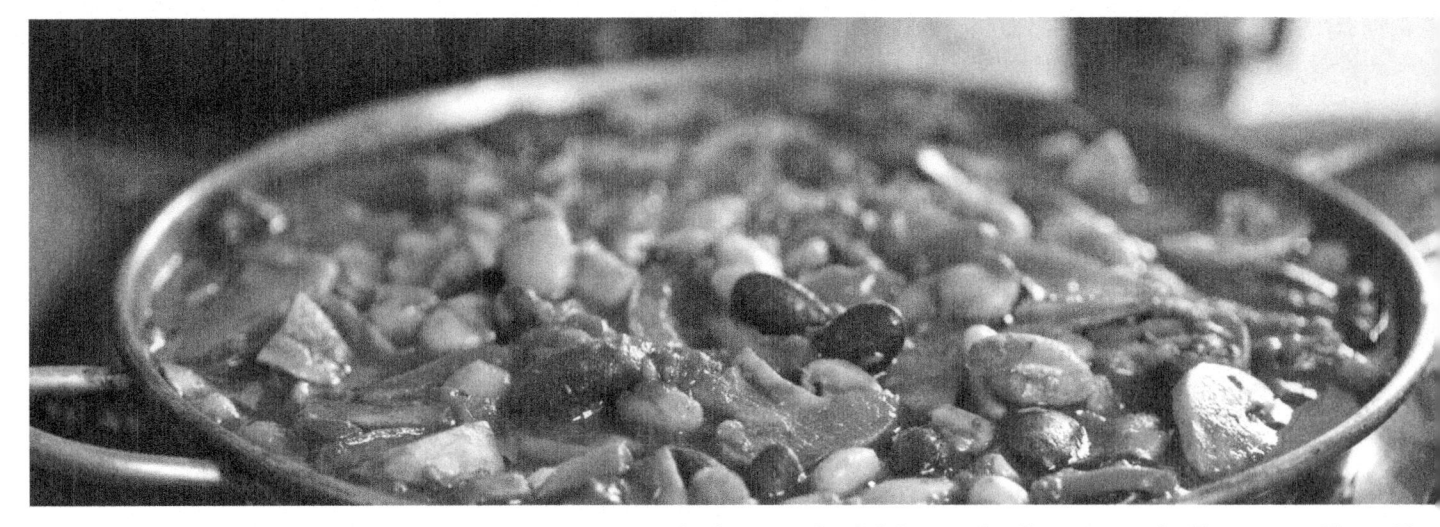

Black bean & vegetable chili with a side salad

This hearty and flavorful black bean and vegetable chili is a perfect dinner option for vegetarians and anyone looking for a healthy and delicious meal. Paired with a simple side salad, this dish is sure to satisfy your hunger and provide essential nutrients.

Serving(s): 04　　　Preparing time: 15 mins　　　Cooking time: 30 mins

Ingredients

- 1 can (15 oz) black beans, drained and rinsed: 0
- 1 can (15 oz) diced tomatoes, with juices: 0
- 1 red bell pepper, diced: 0
- 1 green bell pepper, diced: 0
- 1 medium onion, diced: 0
- 3 cloves garlic, minced: 0
- 1 tbsp chili powder: 0
- 1 tsp ground cumin: 0
- 1/2 tsp paprika: 0
- Salt and black pepper to taste: 0
- 2 tbsp olive oil: 9
- 2 cups mixed greens: 0
- 1/2 cup cherry tomatoes, halved: 0
- 1/4 cup chopped cilantro: 0
- 1/4 cup red onion, thinly sliced: 0
- 1 tbsp balsamic vinegar: 1
- 1 tbsp extra-virgin olive oil: 4

Directions

1. Heat 2 tbsp olive oil in a large saucepan over medium heat. Add diced onion, bell peppers, and garlic. Cook for 5-7 minutes or until softened.
2. Add chili powder, cumin, paprika, salt, and black pepper to the pan. Stir well to combine and cook for another minute.
3. Add diced tomatoes and their juices, along with 1 cup of water to the pan. Bring to a boil, then reduce heat and le simmer for 15-20 minutes.
4. Add the drained and rinsed black beans to the pan and cook for an additional 5 minutes, or until heated through.
5. While the chili is cooking, prepare the side salad. In a large bowl, combine mixed greens, cherry tomatoes, cilantro, and red onion. Toss with balsamic vinegar and extra-virgin olive oil.
6. Serve the chili hot, topped with fresh cilantro and with the side salad on the side.

NUTRITIONS (PER SERVING)

Calories: 300　　Protein: 14g　　Fat: 10g　　Carbohydrates: 40g　　Fiber: 14g　　Sugar: 9g

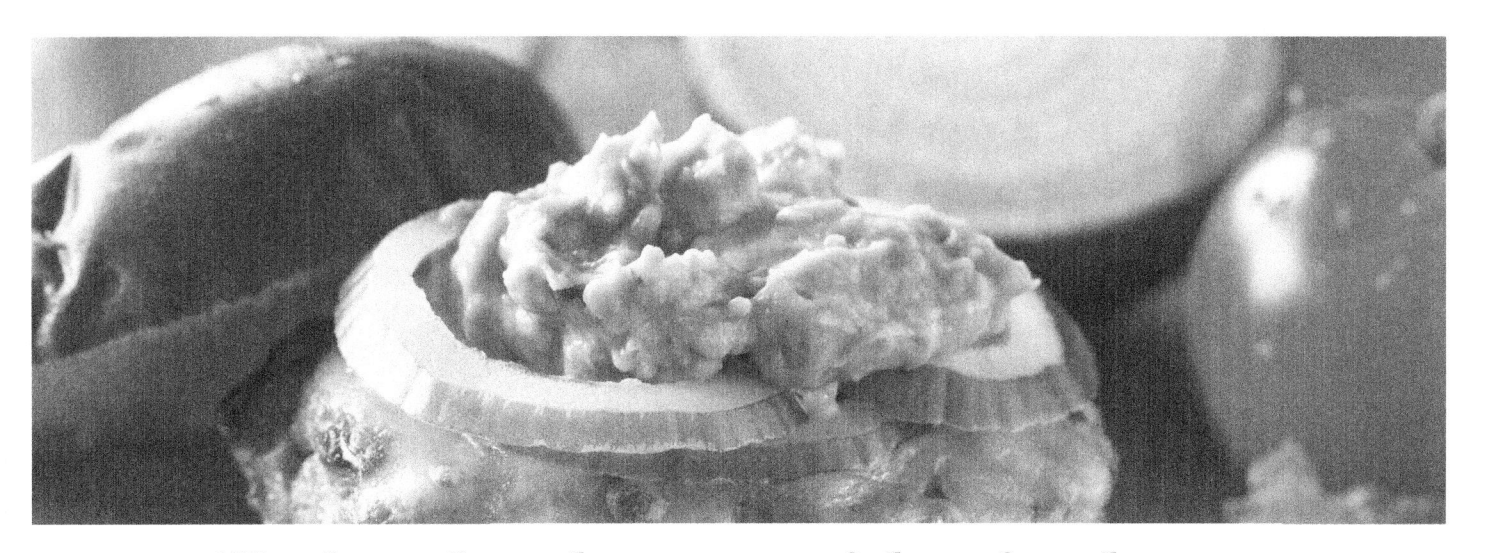

Grilled turkey burger with mixed greens & avocado slices 7

For those who are looking for a healthy and tasty lunch option, this grilled turkey burger with mixed greens and avocado slices is a great choice. It's high in protein and fiber, and packed with nutritious veggies and healthy fats. It's also quick and easy to prepare, making it perfect for busy weekdays.

Serving(s): 04　　　Preparing time: 15 mins　　　Cooking time: 12 mins

Ingredients

- 1 lb ground turkey: 0 SmartPoints
- 1/2 cup finely chopped onion: 0 SmartPoints
- 2 cloves garlic, minced: 0 SmartPoints
- 1 egg, beaten: 0 SmartPoints
- 1/4 cup whole wheat breadcrumbs: 2 SmartPoints
- 1 tsp salt: 0 SmartPoints
- 1/2 tsp black pepper: 0 SmartPoints
- 4 whole grain burger buns: 16 SmartPoints
- 2 cups mixed greens: 0 SmartPoints
- 1 avocado, sliced: 9 SmartPoints

Directions

1. In a large bowl, mix together the ground turkey, onion, garlic, beaten egg, breadcrumbs, salt, and pepper until well combined.
2. Divide the mixture into four equal portions and shape each portion into a patty.
3. Preheat a grill or grill pan over medium-high heat. Grill the turkey burgers for about 5-6 minutes on each side, or until cooked through.
4. Toast the burger buns, if desired.
5. To assemble the burgers, place a turkey patty on the bottom half of each bun. Top with mixed greens and sliced avocado. Cover with the top half of the bun.
6. Serve and enjoy!

NUTRITIONS (PER SERVING)

Calories: 390　　Protein: 32g　　Fat: 19g　　Carbohydrates: 43g　　Fiber: 7g　　Sodium: 720mg

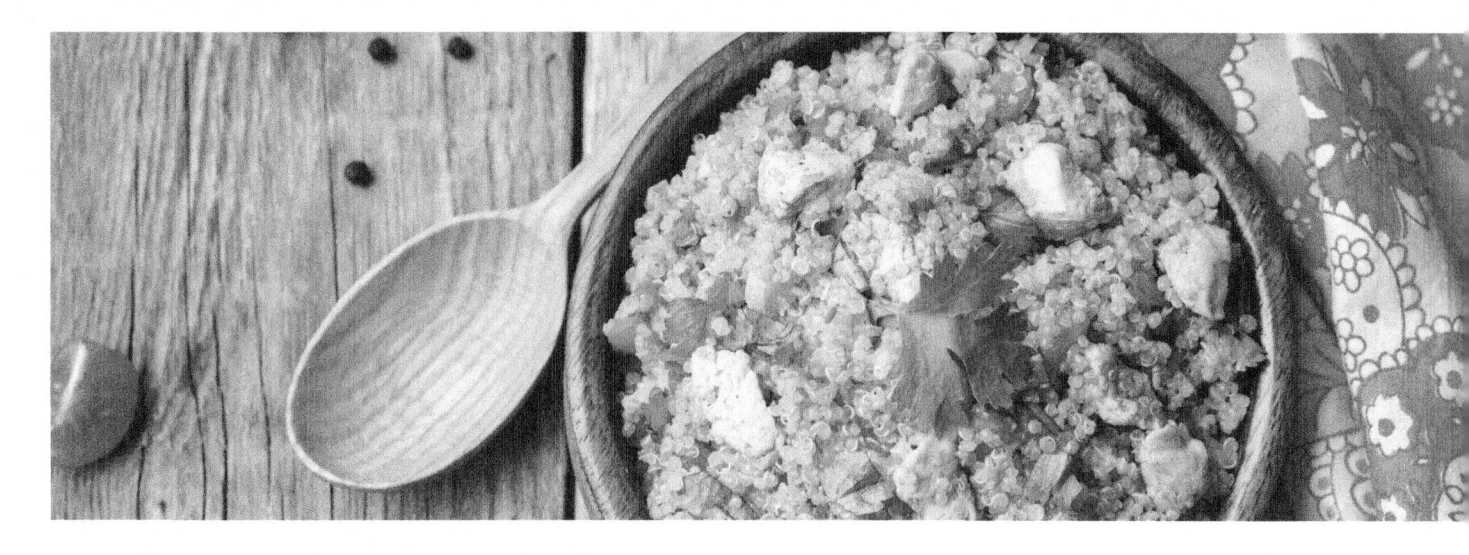

Baked tilapia with quinoa & roasted vegetables

This baked tilapia with quinoa and roasted vegetables is a delicious and healthy lunch option that is easy to prepare. Tilapia is a low-fat, high-protein fish that is rich in essential nutrients, while quinoa is a great source of fiber and protein. The roasted vegetables add flavor and nutrition to the dish.

Serving(s): 04   Preparing time: 10 mins   Cooking time: 20-24 mins

Ingredients

- 4 tilapia fillets
- 2 cups cooked quinoa
- 2 cups mixed vegetables, chopped (such as bell peppers, zucchini, and onion)
- 2 tbsp olive oil
- 1/2 tsp garlic powder
- 1/2 tsp onion powder
- Salt and pepper, to taste

Directions

1. Preheat the oven to 400°F (200°C).
2. Season the tilapia fillets with garlic powder, onion powder, salt, and pepper.
3. Place the tilapia fillets in a baking dish and bake for 10-12 minutes, or until cooked through.
4. While the tilapia is baking, toss the mixed vegetables with olive oil, salt, and pepper. Spread the vegetables out on a baking sheet and roast in the oven for 10-12 minutes, or until tender and lightly browned.
5. Serve the baked tilapia with cooked quinoa and roasted vegetables on the side.

NUTRITIONS (PER SERVING)

Calories: 360   Protein: 37g   Fat: 10g   Carbohydrates: 30g   Fiber: 6g   Sodium: 180mg

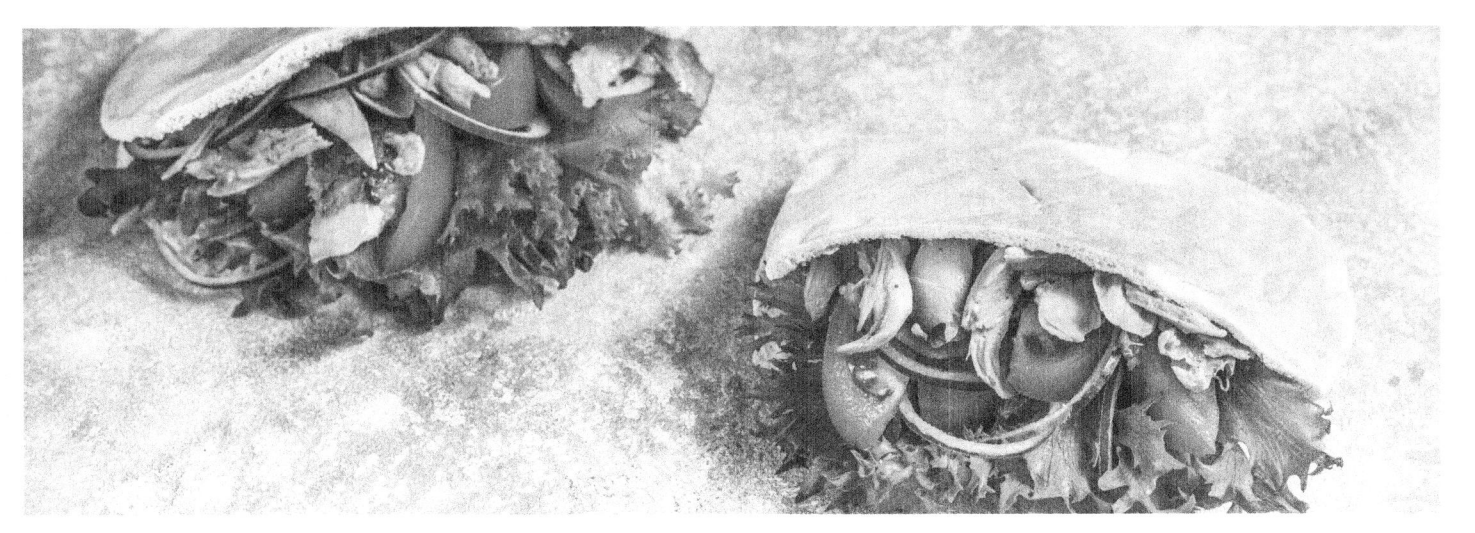

Greek salad with grilled chicken & whole grain pita bread

This Greek salad is a healthy and delicious meal that's perfect for lunch or dinner. With plenty of fresh vegetables and grilled chicken for protein, it's a filling and satisfying dish. The whole grain pita bread is a great addition, providing some healthy carbohydrates to keep you energized.

Serving(s): 04   **Preparing time:** 10 mins   **Cooking time:** 20-24 mins

Ingredients

- 2 boneless, skinless chicken breasts
- 2 tbsp olive oil, divided
- 1 tsp dried oregano
- 1/2 tsp garlic powder
- Salt and black pepper, to taste
- 4 cups mixed greens
- 1/2 red onion, sliced
- 1/2 cucumber, sliced
- 1/2 red bell pepper, sliced
- 1/4 cup kalamata olives
- 2 oz feta cheese, crumbled
- 2 whole grain pita breads

Directions

1. Preheat grill to medium-high heat.
2. In a small bowl, mix together 1 tablespoon olive oil, oregano, garlic powder, salt, and black pepper.
3. Brush the chicken breasts with the oil mixture on both sides.
4. Grill the chicken for 6-7 minutes per side or until cooked through.
5. Remove the chicken from the grill and let it rest for 5 minutes before slicing it into strips.
6. In a large bowl, combine mixed greens, red onion, cucumber, red bell pepper, and kalamata olives.
7. Drizzle the remaining 1 tablespoon of olive oil over the salad and toss to combine.
8. Divide the salad between two plates.
9. Top each plate with sliced chicken, crumbled feta cheese, and a whole grain pita bread on the side.

NUTRITIONS (PER SERVING)

Calories: 479   Protein: 44g   Fat: 22g   Carbohydrates: 28g   Fiber: 7g   Sugar: 6g

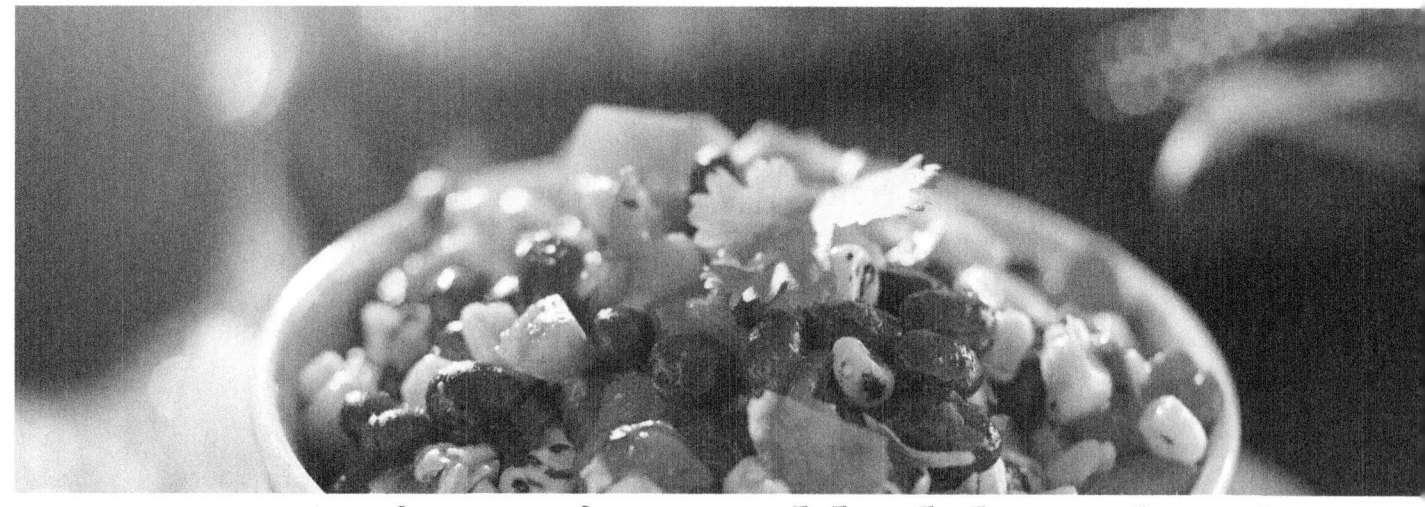

Vegetarian quinoa & black bean bowl with avocado & salsa 5

This vegetarian quinoa and black bean bowl is a delicious and nutritious meal that is packed with protein and fiber. Topped with creamy avocado and tangy salsa, this bowl is a great option for a healthy lunch or dinner.

Serving(s): 04 **Preparing time: 10 mins** **Cooking time: 20 mins**

Ingredients

- 1 cup quinoa, rinsed: 5
- 2 cups water: 0
- 1 can black beans, drained and rinsed: 2
- 1 red bell pepper, diced: 1
- 1 avocado, diced: 7
- 1/4 cup fresh cilantro, chopped: 2
- 1/4 cup salsa: 1
- Salt and pepper, to taste: 0

Directions

1. In a medium saucepan, combine the quinoa and water. Bring to a boil over high heat, then reduce the heat to low and cover. Simmer for 15-20 minutes, or until the water is absorbed and the quinoa is tender.
2. In a large mixing bowl, combine the cooked quinoa, black beans, and red bell pepper. Stir to combine.
3. In a small mixing bowl, mash the avocado with a fork. Season with salt and pepper to taste.
4. Divide the quinoa mixture between four bowls. Top each bowl with diced avocado, fresh cilantro, and salsa. Serve immediately.

NUTRITIONS (PER SERVING)

Calories: 346   Protein: 13g   Fat: 15g   Carbohydrates: 46g   Fiber: 12g   Sugar: 2g

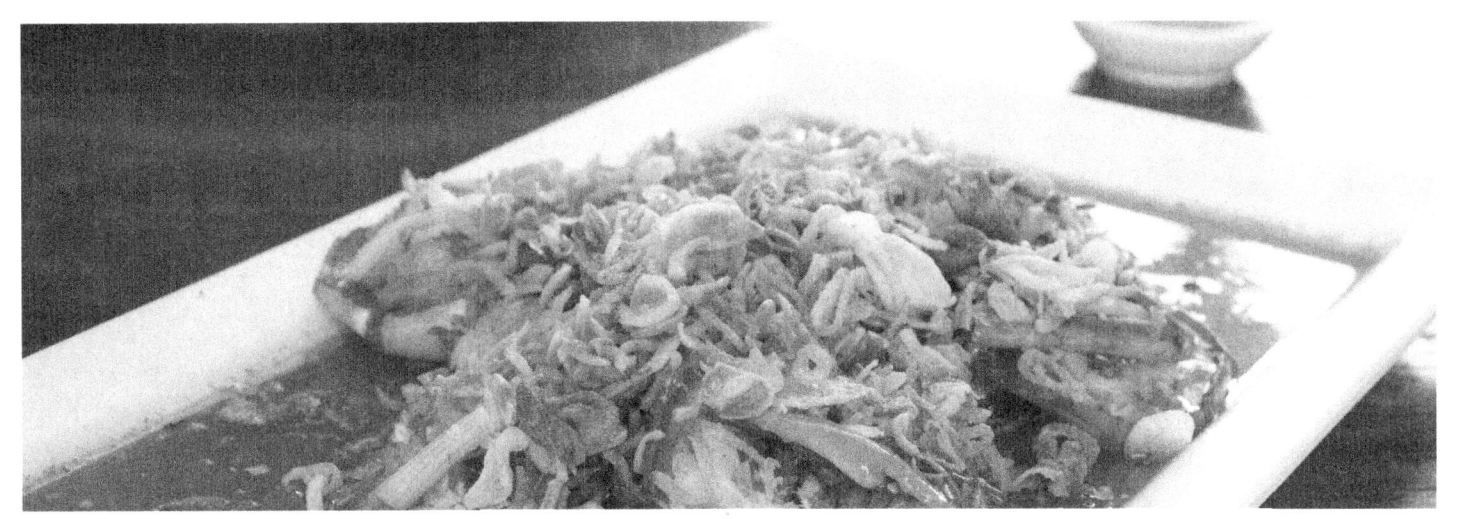

Spicy grilled shrimp with mixed greens & tomato salad [12]

This spicy grilled shrimp salad is a light and refreshing meal that is perfect for a summer lunch or dinner. The combination of juicy shrimp and tangy tomatoes is complemented by a spicy marinade and mixed greens.

Serving(s): 04 **Preparing time: 15 mins** **Cooking time: 6 mins**

Ingredients

- 1 lb large shrimp, peeled and deveined: 0
- 2 tbsp olive oil: 9
- 2 tbsp lime juice: 0
- 1 tbsp honey: 3
- 1 tbsp chili powder: 0
- 1 tsp garlic powder: 0
- 1/2 tsp cumin: 0
- Salt and pepper, to taste: 0
- 6 cups mixed greens: 0
- 2 cups cherry tomatoes, halved: 0
- 1/2 red onion, thinly sliced: 0

Directions

1. Preheat the grill to medium-high heat.
2. In a small mixing bowl, whisk together the olive oil, lime juice, honey, chili powder, garlic powder, cumin, salt, and pepper.
3. Thread the shrimp onto skewers and brush with the marinade.
4. Grill the shrimp for 2-3 minutes per side, or until cooked through.
5. In a large mixing bowl, combine the mixed greens, cherry tomatoes, and red onion. Toss to combine.
6. Divide the salad between four plates. Top each plate with grilled shrimp. Serve immediately.

NUTRITIONS (PER SERVING)

Calories: 220 Protein: 22g Fat: 9g Carbohydrates: 15g Fiber: 3g Sugar: 9g

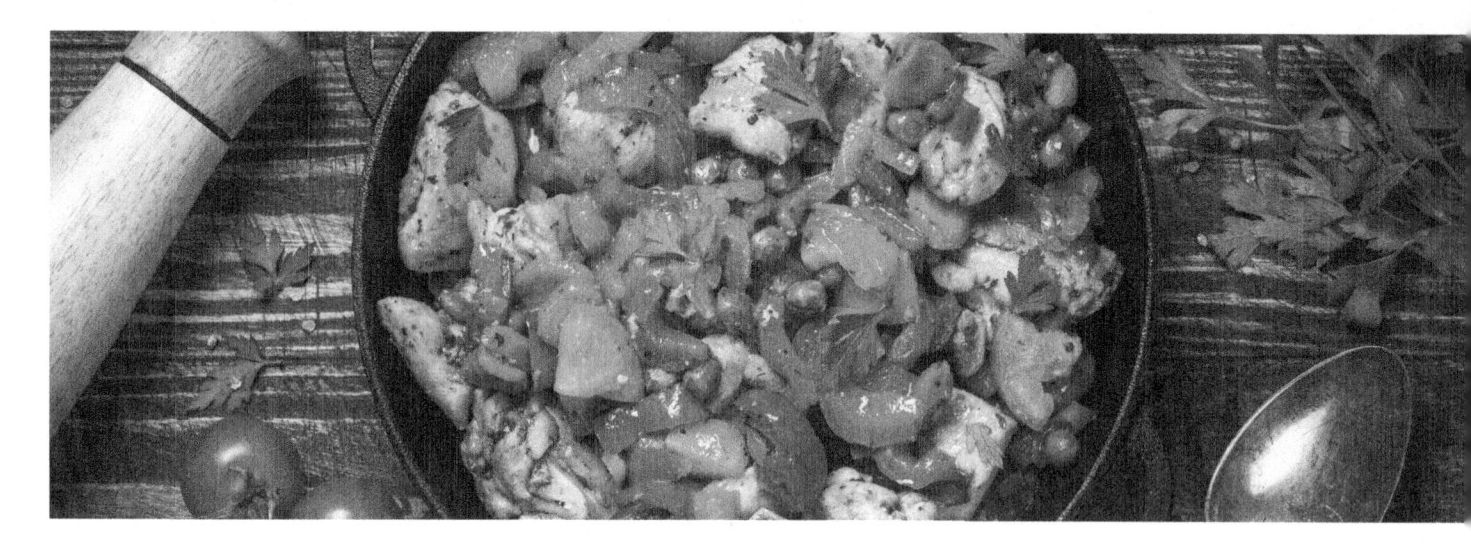

Turkey & vegetable stir-fry with brown rice

This healthy and flavorful stir-fry is loaded with lean turkey, crunchy vegetables, and brown rice for a filling and satisfying meal.

Serving(s): 04 **Preparing time: 10 mins** **Cooking time: 20 mins**

Ingredients

- 1 lb. ground turkey: 4
- 2 cups mixed vegetables (such as broccoli, bell peppers, onions, and carrots): 2
- 1 garlic clove, minced: 0
- 2 tbsp. low-sodium soy sauce: 1
- 1 tbsp. sesame oil: 6
- 1 tsp. honey: 1
- 2 cups cooked brown rice: 4

Directions

1. Heat the sesame oil in a large skillet over medium heat.
2. Add the garlic and sauté for 30 seconds, then add the ground turkey and cook until browned.
3. Add the mixed vegetables and continue to cook for 5-7 minutes, or until tender.
4. In a small bowl, whisk together the soy sauce and honey, then pour over the stir-fry mixture and stir to combine.
5. Serve over cooked brown rice.

NUTRITIONS (PER SERVING)

Calories: 415   Protein: 30g   Fat: 12g   Carbohydrates: 45g   Fiber: 6g   Sugar: 6g

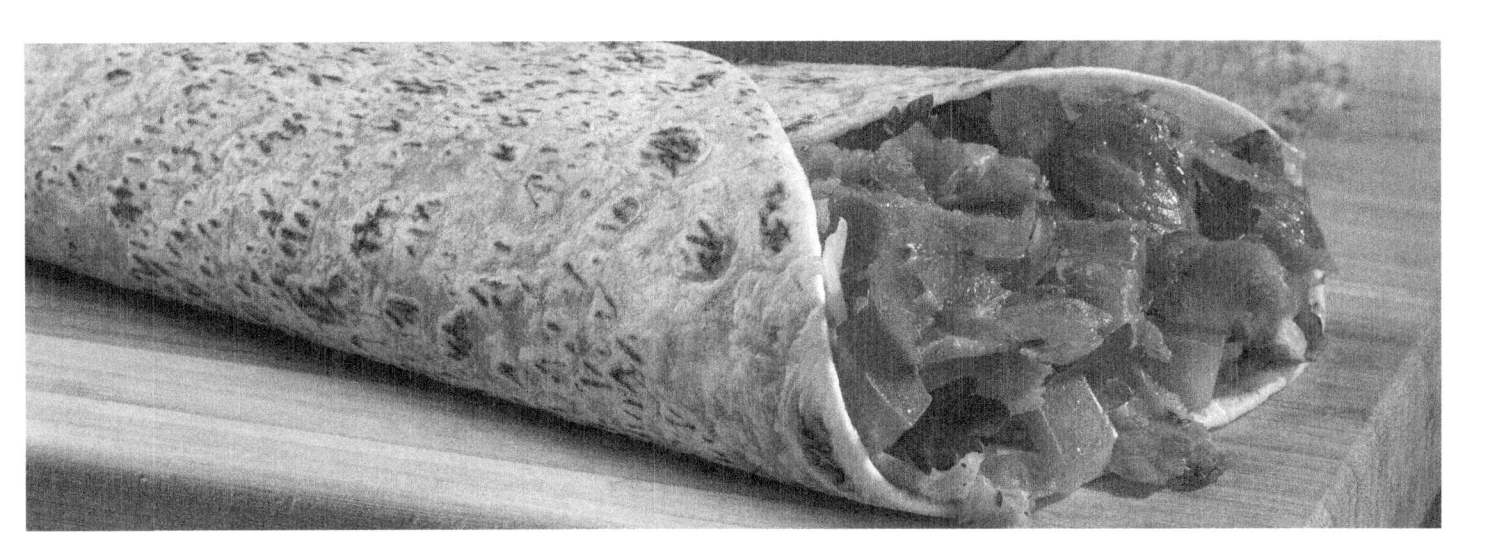

Roasted vegetable & hummus wrap with mixed greens [8]

This vegetarian wrap is packed with roasted veggies, creamy hummus, and fresh greens for a delicious and nutritious meal.

Serving(s): 04 **Preparing time: 10 mins** **Cooking time: 25 mins**

Ingredients

- 1 cup mixed vegetables (such as bell peppers, zucchini, and eggplant): 1
- 1 tbsp. olive oil: 4
- Salt and pepper, to taste: 0
- 1 whole grain wrap: 2
- 1 tbsp. hummus: 1
- 1/2 cup mixed greens: 0

Directions

1. Preheat the oven to 400°F.
2. Toss the mixed vegetables with olive oil and season with salt and pepper.
3. Spread the vegetables out on a baking sheet and roast for 20-25 minutes, or until tender.
4. Warm the whole grain wraps in the microwave for 10-15 seconds.
5. Spread 1 tbsp. of hummus onto each wrap, then add a handful of mixed greens.
6. Top with the roasted vegetables and wrap tightly.

NUTRITIONS (PER SERVING)

Calories: 310   Protein: 9g   Fat: 12g   Carbohydrates: 44g   Fiber: 10g   Sugar: 5g

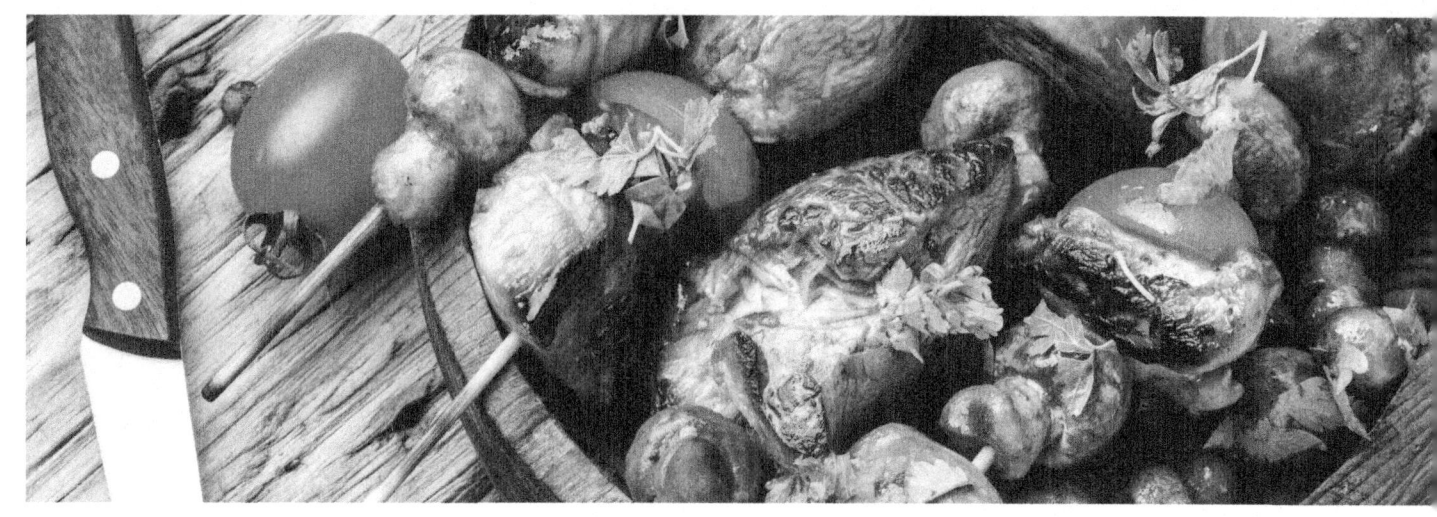

Grilled chicken & vegetable kabobs with brown rice 7

These grilled chicken and vegetable kabobs with brown rice are a flavorful and healthy dinner option. With colorful veggies and juicy chicken, they are a tasty way to get your daily dose of protein and vegetables. Pair them with brown rice for a satisfying and nutritious meal.

Serving(s): 04	Preparing time: 15 mins	Cooking time: 10-12 mins

Ingredients

- 2 large chicken breasts, cut into bite-sized pieces: 5
- 2 bell peppers, cut into chunks: 1
- 1 red onion, cut into chunks: 1
- 8-10 cherry tomatoes: 0
- 1/4 cup olive oil: 8
- 1/4 cup lemon juice: 2
- 1 teaspoon dried oregano: 0
- 1 teaspoon garlic powder: 0
- Salt and pepper, to taste: 0
- 2 cups cooked brown rice: 5

Directions

1. Preheat grill to medium-high heat.
2. In a large bowl, whisk together olive oil, lemon juice, oregano, garlic powder, salt, and pepper.
3. Add chicken pieces, peppers, onion, and cherry tomatoes to the bowl and toss to coat with the marinade.
4. Thread chicken and vegetables onto skewers, alternating between chicken and veggies.
5. Grill kabobs for 10-12 minutes, turning occasionally, until chicken is cooked through and vegetables are tender and lightly charred.
6. Serve kabobs over cooked brown rice.

NUTRITIONS (PER SERVING)

Calories: 350   Protein: 29g   Fat: 10g   Carbohydrates: 38g   Fiber: 5g   Sugar: 6g

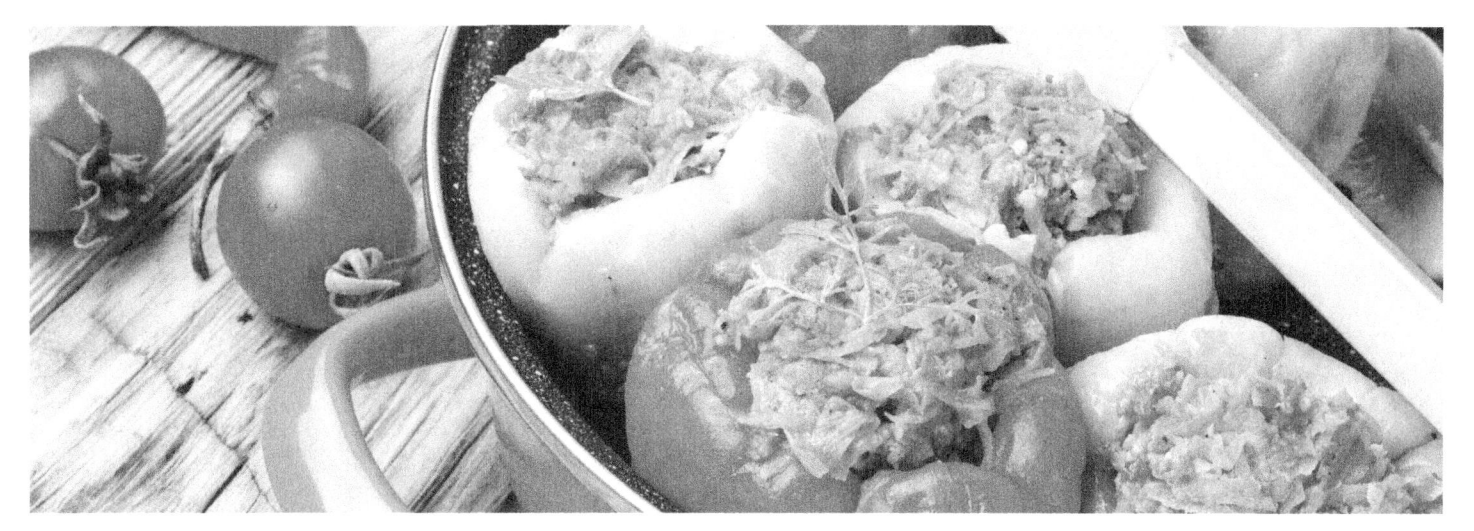

Quinoa & vegetable stuffed bell peppers

These quinoa and vegetable stuffed bell peppers are a colorful and healthy dinner option. They are packed with protein from the quinoa and black beans, and filled with colorful veggies like corn, tomatoes, and peppers. Top with avocado and salsa for a satisfying and nutritious meal.

Serving(s): 04 **Preparing time: 20 mins** **Cooking time: 40-45 mins**

Ingredients

- 4 large bell peppers: 0
- 1 cup cooked quinoa: 5
- 1 can black beans, drained and rinsed: 2
- 1 cup corn: 2
- 1 cup cherry tomatoes, halved: 1
- 1/4 cup chopped fresh cilantro: 1
- 1 tablespoon olive oil: 4
- 1 tablespoon lime juice: 0
- Salt and pepper, to taste: 0
- 1 avocado, diced: 7
- 1/2 cup salsa: 1

Directions

1. Preheat oven to 375°F (190°C).
2. Cut the tops off the bell peppers and remove the seeds and membranes.
3. In a large bowl, mix together the cooked quinoa, black beans, corn, cherry tomatoes, cilantro, olive oil, lime juice, salt, and pepper.
4. Stuff the quinoa mixture into each bell pepper, packing it down firmly.
5. Place the stuffed peppers in a baking dish and cover with foil.
6. Bake for 40-45 minutes, or until the peppers are tender and the filling is heated through.
7. Top each pepper with diced avocado and serve with salsa on the side.

NUTRITIONS (PER SERVING)

Calories: 310   Protein: 11g   Fat: 13g   Carbohydrates: 41g   Fiber: 13g   Sugar: 9g

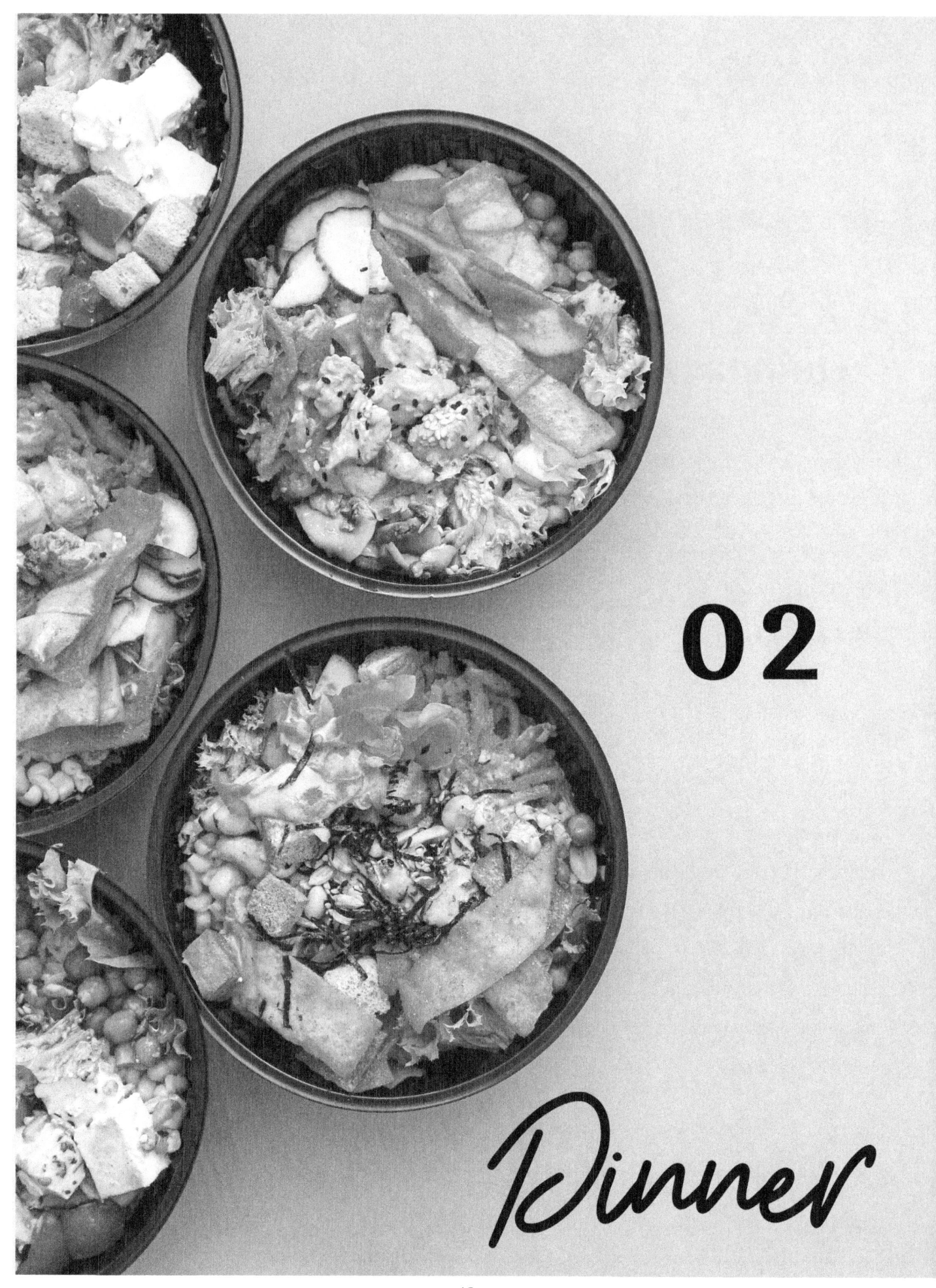

02

Dinner

GRILLED SHRIMP PANZANELLA SKEWERS

1

NUTRITION:
Per Serving: Calories: 216kcal, Carbohydrates: 18g, Protein: 28g, Fat: 3g, Saturated Fat: 1g, Cholesterol: 188mg, Sodium: 376mg Fiber: 2.5g, Sugar: 7g

INGREDIENTS

- 32 jumbo peeled shrimp, 18 oz total
- ½ tsp kosher salt
- 2 large peaches
- 1 cup grape tomatoes
- 1 thick slice sourdough bread, cut into 3/4-inch cubes (2 oz)
- 16 long wooden or metal skewers
- Cooking spray
- 1 handful fresh basil leaves
- Balsamic vinegar or glaze, for serving

DIRECTION

1. Pat the shrimp dry and season both sides with salt.
2. Cut the peaches into thick wedges (6 to 8 per peach, depending on size).
3. If using large tomatoes, core them and cut them into wedges approximately the same size.
4. Thread the shrimp, peaches, tomatoes, and cubed bread onto doubled skewers, alternating as you like but beginning and ending each skewer with shrimp, for a total of 8 kabobs. Lightly spray with cooking oil.
5. Preheat the grill with high heat and oil the grates.
6. Grill the kabobs for 2 to 3 minutes per side, until the shrimp are pink and firm and the bread is lightly charred. The tomatoes may be bursting.
7. To serve, place the kabobs on a platter. Thinly slice or tear the basil and sprinkle it over everything with a drizzle of balsamic vinegar.

GROUND TURKEY SKILLET WITH ZUCCHINI, CORN, BLACK BEANS

5

NUTRITION:
Calories: 266kcal, Carbohydrates: 22.5g, Protein: 28g, Fat: 8.5g, Saturated Fat: 2.5g, Cholesterol: 80mg, Sodium: 525mg, Fiber: 6.5g, Sugar: 4g

INGREDIENTS

- 14 ounces zucchini, quartered, sliced 3/4 inch
- 1 pound 93% lean ground turkey
- 1/4 cup chopped onion
- 1 tablespoon tomato paste
- 3/4 cups canned black beans, rinsed & drained, 1 large diced tomato
- 3/4 cups corn kernels, fresh or frozen
- 1 jalapeño, diced
- 1 cloves garlic, minced
- 2 tbsp chopped cilantro, plus more for garnish
- 1 1/4 teaspoon cumin
- 1 1/4 teaspoon kosher salt
- 1/4 cup water, lime wedges

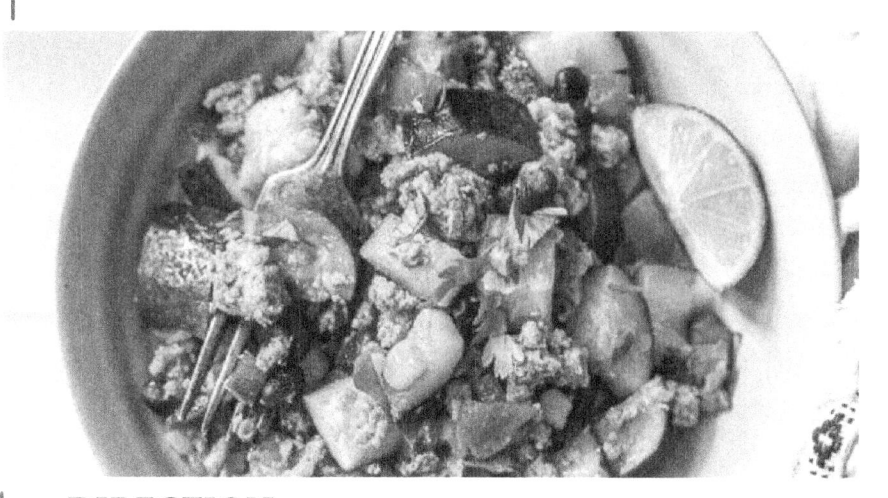

DIRECTION

1. Spray a large skillet over high heat with oil and brown the turkey, season with 1 teaspoon salt and 1 teaspoon cumin.
2. Cook breaking the meat up until the turkey is cooked through, about 5 minutes.
3. Push the meat to the side, add the onion and tomato paste and cook 1 minute.
4. Add the black beans, corn, tomato, jalapeño pepper, garlic, cilantro and corn and stir with 1/4 cup water.
5. Add the zucchini remaining 1/4 teaspoon salt and cumin.
6. Mix and cover, cook low 4 to 5 minutes or until the zucchini is tender crisp.
7. Serve with lime wedges and more cilantro if desired.

GRILLED BRUSCHETTA CHICKEN `3`

NUTRITION:
Calories: 282kcal, Carbohydrates: 7g, Protein: 38.5g, Fat: 11g, Saturated Fat: 3.5g, Cholesterol: 116mg, Sodium: 173mg, Fiber: 1.5g, Sugar: 0.5g

INGREDIENTS
- 3 medium vine ripe tomatoes
- 2 small cloves garlic, minced
- 1/4 cup chopped red onion
- 2 tbsp fresh basil leaves, chopped
- 1 tbsp extra virgin oil
- 1 tbsp balsamic vinegar
- kosher salt and fresh cracked pepper to taste
- 3 oz part skim mozzarella, diced (omit for whole30, paleo)
- 1.25 lbs 8 thin sliced chicken cutlets

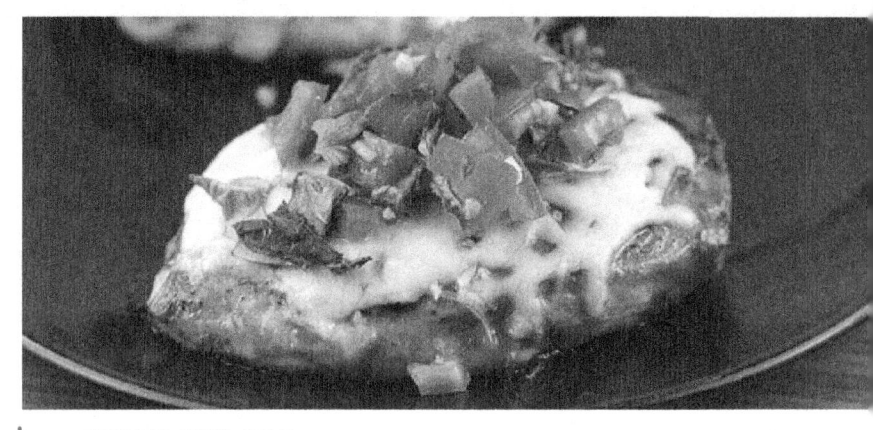

DIRECTION
1. Combine onion, olive oil, balsamic, 1/4 tsp kosher salt and pepper. Set aside a few minutes.
2. Chop tomatoes and place in a large bowl. Combine with garlic, basil, onion-balsamic combo and additional 1/8 tsp salt and pepper to taste. Set aside and let it sit at least 10 minutes or as long as overnight.
3. Toss in the cheese when ready to serve.
4. Season chicken with salt and fresh pepper.
5. Preheat the grill to medium-high, clean and oil the grates to prevent sticking.
6. Grill the chicken 2 minutes on each side, set aside on a platter and top with bruschetta and serve.

GRILLED FLANK STEAK WITH BLACK BEAN AND CORN SALSA `4`

NUTRITION:
Calories: 250kcal, Carbohydrates: 9g, Protein: 25.5g, Fat: 9.5g, Sodium: 385mg, Fiber: 2.5g, Sugar: 2.5g

INGREDIENTS
- 1 1/2 lb flank steak
- 1/2 tsp cumin
- 2 garlic cloves, crushed
- 1/2 tsp kosher salt
- fresh cracked pepper to taste

For the black bean, corn and tomatoes:
- 3 tbsp red onion, minced
- 1 tsp olive oil
- 1/4 cup fresh squeezed lime juice
- 2 medium vine ripe tomatoes, diced
- 1 cup canned black beans, drained and rinsed
- 1 cups frozen corn kernels, fresh is fine
- 2 tbsp finely minced cilantro
- kosher salt and fresh pepper to taste

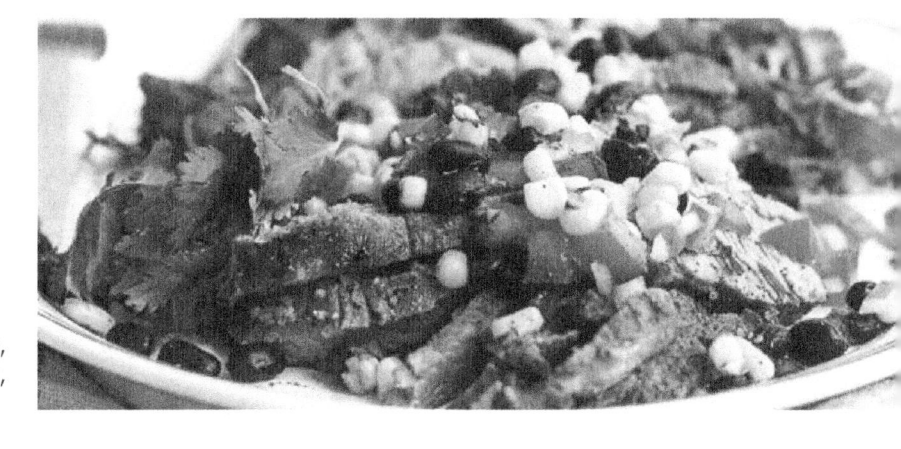

DIRECTION
1. Season the steak: Season the flank steak with the crushed garlic, cumin, salt and pepper and set aside 5-10 minutes.
2. Make the salsa: Meanwhile, combine red onions, olive oil, lime juice, salt and pepper in a medium bowl and set aside a few minutes.
3. Add tomatoes, black beans, corn, cilantro and set aside.
4. Preheat the grill. Heat a clean lightly greased indoor or outdoor grill on high heat.
5. Grill the steak on high heat, 6-8 minutes on each side or until your desired degree of done-ness. Until a probe thermometer inserted into the thickest part of the steak registers 130F to 135°F for medium to medium rare
6. Let the meat rest about 5 minutes before slicing.
7. Slice the beef into thin slices across the grain, place on a platter and top with corn, black bean and tomato salad.

AIR FRYER CHICKEN SANDWICH WITH SRIRACHA MAYO

NUTRITION:
Calories: 334kcal, Carbohydrates: 31g, Protein: 35g, Fat: 8g, Saturated Fat: 1.5g, Cholesterol: 100mg, Sodium: 796mg, Fiber: 6g, Sugar: 7g

INGREDIENTS

- 2 boneless, skinless chicken breasts, 16 ounces
- 1 cup 1% buttermilk
- 1 cup pickle juice
- 1 large egg, beaten
- Kosher salt
- 1/2 cup all purpose flour
- 1/2 teaspoon garlic powder
- 1/2 teaspoon paprika
- 1/8 teaspoon cayenne pepper
- olive oil spray
- 4 tablespoons light mayo
- 1 tablespoon sriracha
- 12 dill pickle chips
- 4 whole wheat potato rolls, such as Martins

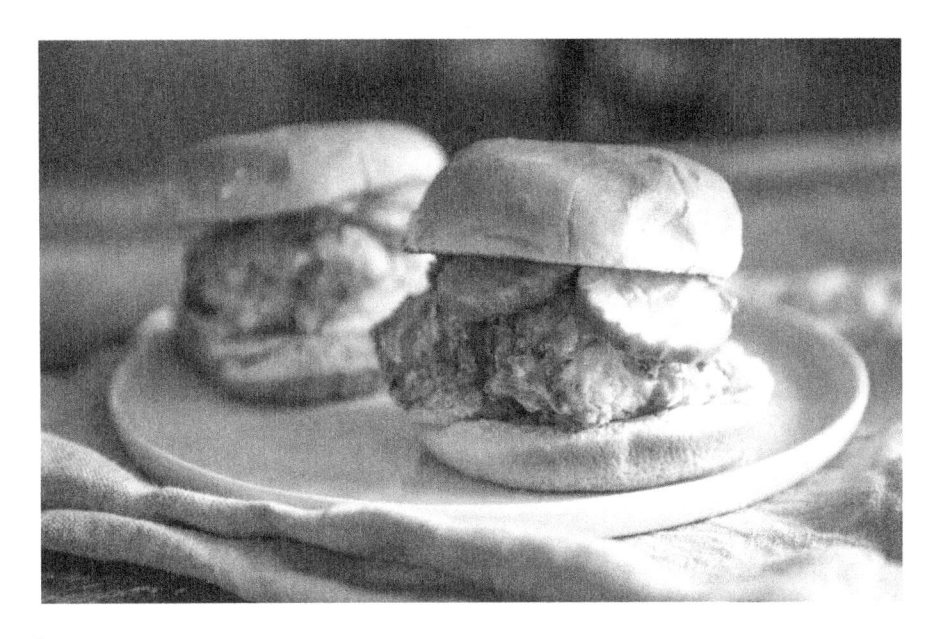

DIRECTION

1. Pound out the thicker end of the chicken breast to make the thickness even on both ends, about 1/2-inch thick, this will ensure the chicken cooks even, then cut each breast in half to make 4 pieces.
2. Whisk buttermilk and pickle juice in a bowl.
3. Add chicken and toss to coat; cover with plastic wrap and chill at least 6 hours or overnight.
4. Combine flour, garlic powder, paprika, 1/2 teaspoon salt, and cayenne pepper in a shallow bowl.
5. Whisk egg in another bowl.
6. Line the air fryer basket with an air fryer parchment liner (these are sold on Amazon, look for parchment with the holes).
7. Working with one chicken breast at a time, dip chicken in flour mixture, shaking off excess. Then into the egg and back into the flour, using the back of a fork to coat well so it adheres.
8. Shake excess then transfer to the prepared air fryer basket and spray tops with oil.
9. Air fry in batches as needed 380F until golden and cooked through, about 15 to 18 minutes, turning halfway depending on the thickness, or until an instant-read thermometer inserted into the thickest part of the breast reads 165°F.
10. To assemble sandwiches, place the mayo on the top of rolls, place the chicken on the bottom roll followed by the pickle chips and tops of rolls.

SKILLET CAJUN SPICED FISH WITH TOMATOES 0

NUTRITION:
Calories: 206kcal, Carbohydrates: 10g, Protein: 33g, Fat: 4g, Sodium: 341mg Fiber: 2g, Sugar: 0.5g

INGREDIENTS

- 1 tsp olive oil
- 4 6 ounce pieces white fish fillets (flounder, fluke, tilapia)
- 3/4 cup onion, chopped
- 2 cloves garlic, minced
- 3/4 cup diced green bell pepper
- 2 1/2 cups tomatoes, chopped
- 1 tbsp Cajun spice seasoning

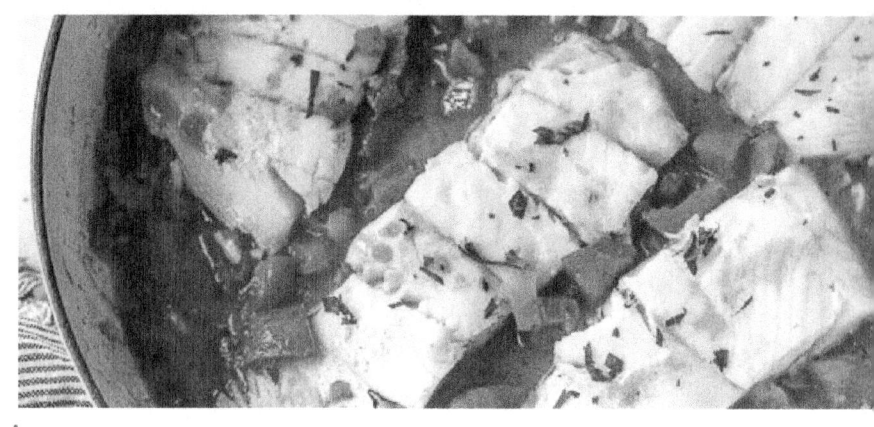

DIRECTION

1. In a deep skillet, cook onion and garlic in olive oil on medium heat for a few minutes until soft.
2. Add tomatoes, peppers and spices, stir and cook until tomatoes are soft, about 2-3 minutes.
3. Lay fish fillets in the sauce, cover and cook on medium-low until fish flakes easily, approx 12-15.
4. To serve, place fish on plate and spoon sauce on top. Serve immediately.

SALMON FRIED RICE
4

NUTRITION:
Calories: 408kcal, Carbohydrates: 28g, Protein: 34g, Fat: 17.5g, Saturated Fat: 3.5g, Cholesterol: 248.5mg, Sodium: 733mg Fiber: 4g, Sugar: 2.5g

INGREDIENTS

- 4 ounces wild salmon fillet, skinned
- 1 teaspoon sesame oil, divided
- 1 large or 2 small scallions, thinly sliced, whites and greens separated
- 1/2 cup cooked cold rice, preferably brown short grain
- 3/4 cup frozen cauliflower rice
- 1 large egg, beaten
- 1/2 tablespoon soy sauce, or gluten-free Tamari
- Sriracha or Chile-garlic sauce, optional for serving

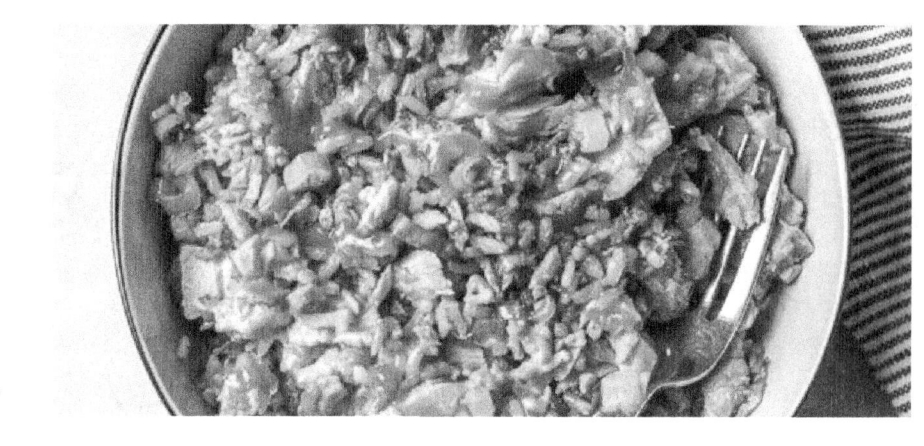

DIRECTION

1. Cook salmon in a skillet over medium-high heat about 5 minutes on each side. Set aside and flake the salmon into small chunks with a fork. Wipe the skillet.
2. Heat 1/2 teaspoon of the oil in a medium nonstick skillet over medium-high. Add scallion whites and cook, stirring, until fragrant, about 1 minute.
3. Add the rice in an even layer. Cook, without stirring, 2 to 3 minutes, or until the bottom becomes slightly crispy. Add the cauliflower rice, continue to cook, stirring occasionally, 2 to 3 minutes, or until combined.
4. With a spoon or spatula, push the rice to one side of the skillet. Crack the egg onto the other side.
5. Cook, constantly stirring the egg, 30 to 60 seconds or until cooked through. Mix the rice, cauliflower and egg to thoroughly combine. Stir in the soy sauce and sesame oil.
6. Gently fold in the reserved salmon and toss, serve immediately garnished with scallion greens. Serve with sriracha sauce, if desired.

CHEESEBURGER CRUNCH WRAP

11

NUTRITION:
Calories: 354kcal, Carbohydrates: 22g, Protein: 33g, Fat: 18.5g, Saturated Fat: 6.5g, Cholesterol: 103.5mg, Sodium: 1282.5mg, Fiber: 10g, Sugar: 1.5g

INGREDIENTS

- 8 ounces 93% ground turkey
- 3/4 teaspoon kosher salt
- 2 large, 10-inch low-carb tortillas (Tumaros)
- 2 slices American or cheddar, (.7 ounces each)
- 2 tablespoons ketchup
- 1 tablespoon golden mustard
- dill pickle and red onion slices
- shredded lettuce
- olive oil spray
- **Optional for crunch:**
- Add air fryer french fries or chips, if desired (extra)

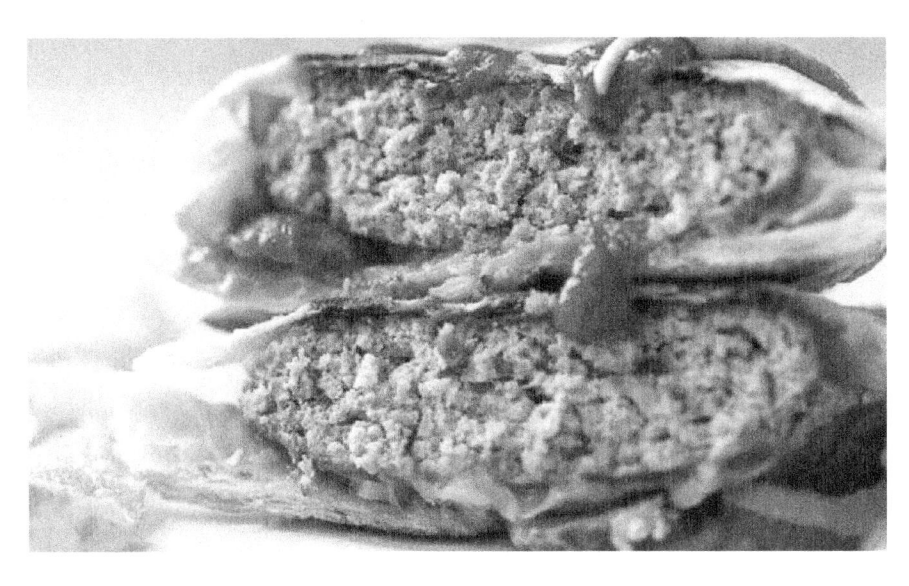

DIRECTION

1. Form meat into two flat patties, 1/3 inch thick. Season with salt.

For Skillet:
1. Spray a skillet and heat over medium heat. Add the burgers and cook 5 minutes on each side, until cooked through.
2. Wipe clean and spray with oil, keep heated over medium-low heat.
3. Place the burger in the center of the wrap followed by the cheese, pickles, onion, ketchup, mustard and lettuce. Fold the sides over to crunch wrap it by folding the sides over each other.
4. Place on the hot skillet, folded side down. Cook until browned, 1 to 2 minutes, then flip and continue cooking until browned and crisp, 1 to 2 minutes more.

For Air Fryer:
1. Air fry the burgers 400F 10 to 14 min turning halfway, until cooked through in the center.
2. Wipe the air fryer basket clean and spray with oil.
3. Place the burger in the center of the wrap followed by the cheese, pickles, onion, ketchup, mustard and lettuce.
4. Fold the sides over to crunch wrap it and place it on the air fryer basket, folded side down.
5. Preheat your air fryer for 5 minutes at 400 degrees F, and then add your wrap inside folded side down, spritz the top with oil and air fry for 4 to 5 minutes, flip carefully halfway.

AIR FRYER BACON WRAPPED PORK TENDERLOIN `3`

NUTRITION:
Calories: 153kcal, Carbohydrates: 0.5g, Protein: 26.5g, Fat: 4g, Saturated Fat: 1.5g, Cholesterol: 76mg, Sodium: 258.5mg

INGREDIENTS
- 1/2 teaspoon kosher salt
- 1/4 teaspoon ground black pepper
- 1 pork tenderloin, about 1 1/2 lbs
- 6 center cut strips bacon
- cooking string

DIRECTION
1. Season pork with salt and pepper. Lay the bacon on a cutting board to be roughly the same size as the tenderloin.
2. Cut two bacon strips in half (since the ends are thinner, they don't need a whole strip). Lay two halves next to each other, then four full strips, then the other two halves next to each other.
3. Carefully lay the tenderloin over the bacon. Tightly roll up the pork jelly-roll style, starting with a long side. Tie the roast at 2-inch intervals with kitchen string each about 12-inches long.
4. Carefully cut the tenderloin in half to fit in the air fryer.
5. Put the tenderloin inside and fry at 400 F for 20 minutes turning halfway, until an instant read thermometer inserted into the center reads 145-150°F. Let the pork rest about 5 minutes before slicing. Slice into 12 slices.

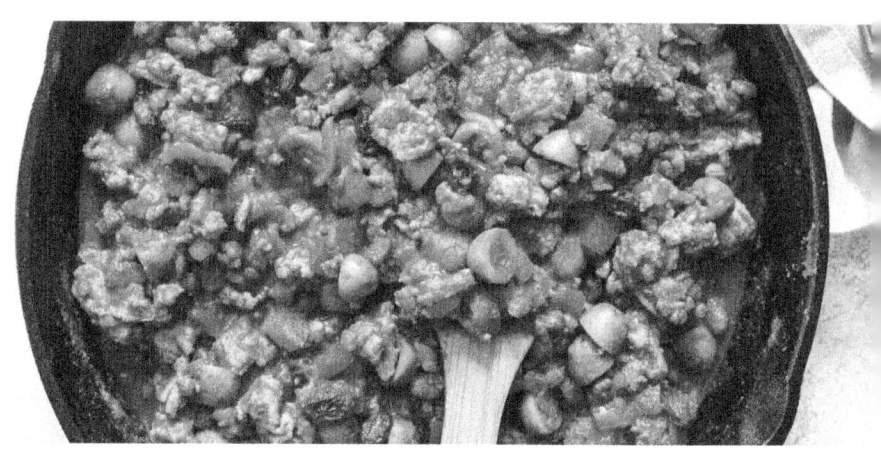

TURKEY PICADILLO
`5`

NUTRITION:
Calories: 238kcal, Carbohydrates: 7.5g, Protein: 29g, Fat: 11g, Saturated Fat: 3g, Cholesterol: 100mg, Sodium: 354mg Fiber: 1.5g, Sugar: 2.5g

INGREDIENTS
- 1.33 lb 93% lean ground turkey
- 4 oz tomato sauce, (1/2 can)
- 1 tsp kosher salt
- 1 tsp ground cumin
- 2 small bay leaves
- 2 tbsp green Spanish pitted olives, plus 2 tbsp brine
- Sofrito:
- 1 medium tomato
- 1/2 medium onion, finely chopped
- 2 cloves minced garlic
- 2 tbsp red bell pepper, finely chopped
- 2 tbsp cilantro, optional

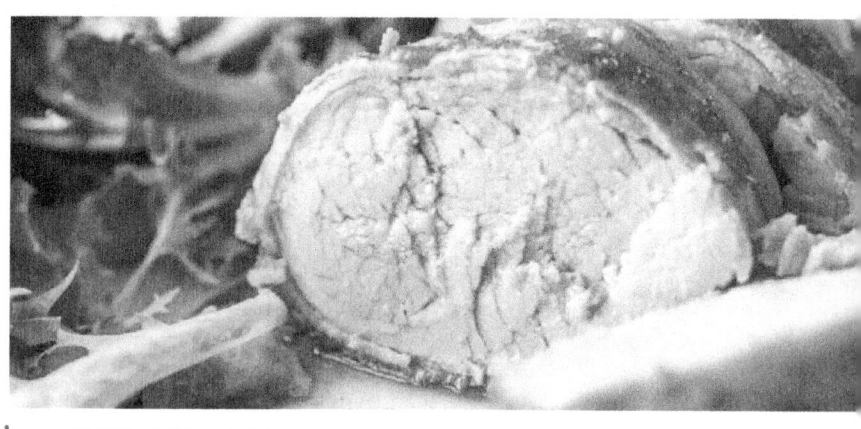

DIRECTION
1. Brown the ground turkey on medium heat in large sauté pan and season with salt and pepper. Use a wooden spoon to break the meat up into small pieces.
2. Meanwhile, while turkey is cooking, make the sofrito by chopping onion, garlic, pepper, tomato and cilantro. (I quickly do it in my mini chopper)
3. Add sofrito to the meat and continue cooking on a low heat.
4. Add olives and about 2 tbsp of the brine (this adds great flavor) cumin, bay leaves, and more salt if needed.
5. Add tomato sauce and 1/4 cup of water and mix well.
6. Reduce heat to low and simmer covered about 15 to 20 minutes to let the flavors meld.

AHI TUNA POKE STACKS

9

NUTRITION:
Calories: 561kcal, Carbohydrates: 37.5g, Protein: 48.5g, Fat: 24.5g, Saturated Fat: 3.5g, Cholesterol: 76mg, Sodium: 1620.5mg, Fiber: 7.5g, Sugar: 5g

INGREDIENTS

For Tuna:
- 12 ounces raw sushi grade tuna, cubed small
- 3 tablespoons reduced sodium soy sauce, or gluten-free tamari, liquid aminos
- 1 1/2 teaspoon sesame oil
- 1 teaspoon sriracha
- 1 scallion, sliced

For Stacks:
- 1 cup cooked short-grain brown rice, heated
- 1 tablespoon rice vinegar
- 1 cup peeled and diced cucumber, about 1 medium
- 1/2 cup mashed avocado, about 1 medium
- 4 teaspoons Furikake, such as Eden Shake or use sesame seeds
- 4 teaspoons reduced-sodium soy sauce, or gluten-free
- 4 teaspoons mayonnaise
- 1 teaspoon sriracha sauce

DIRECTION

1. In a large bowl combine tuna, soy sauce, sesame oil, sriracha and scallions.
2. Gently toss and set aside while you prepare the rest.
3. Place the heated rice in a bowl and add rice vinegar; stir.
4. In a small bowl, combine mayonnaise and sriracha sauce.
5. Lightly spray the inside of a 1 cup dry measuring cup with oil (use one with straight edges) then start by layering 1/4 cup cucumber, then 2 tablespoon of avocado and smooth, then 1/4 of the tuna and flatten with the back of a spoon, and finally 1/4 cup rice.
6. Carefully turn the cup upside down to turn the stack out onto a plate, lightly tapping the bottom of the cup if necessary.
7. Sprinkle with Furikake and drizzle with 1 teaspoon soy sauce and sriracha mayonnaise.
    a. Repeat with remaining ingredients.

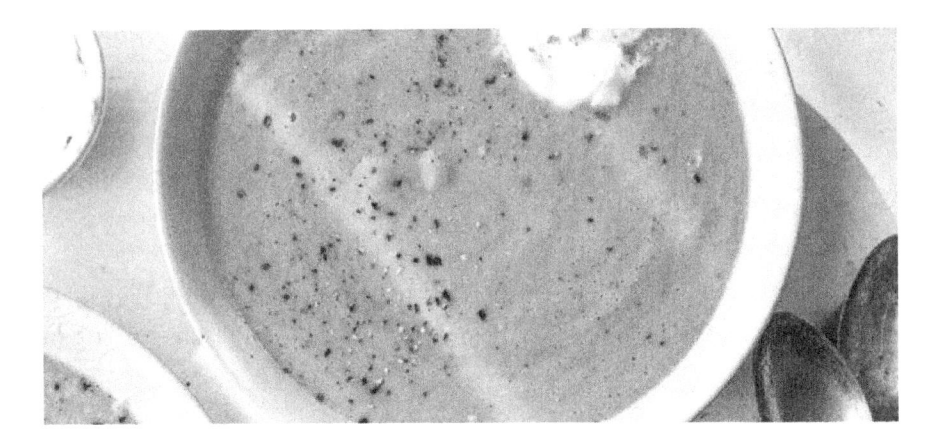

SPRING PEA AND FRESH HERBS SOUP

2

NUTRITION:
Calories: 160kcal, Carbohydrates: 20.5g, Protein: 6.5g, Fat: 6g, Saturated Fat: 1g, Cholesterol: 1.5mg, Sodium: 444mg, Fiber: 6.5g, Sugar: 8.5g

INGREDIENTS

- 1 1/2 tablespoons extra virgin olive oil
- 10 scallions, thinly sliced
- 1 1/2 tablespoons chopped fresh tarragon or basil
- 3 cups fresh or frozen green peas
- 3 cups vegetable broth
- 2 tablespoons chopped fresh mint
- 1 lemon, zested and juice reserved
- 3/4 to 1 teaspoon kosher salt
- 1/4 teaspoon freshly ground black pepper
- 3 tablespoons whole yogurt
- 1/4 teaspoon ground coriander

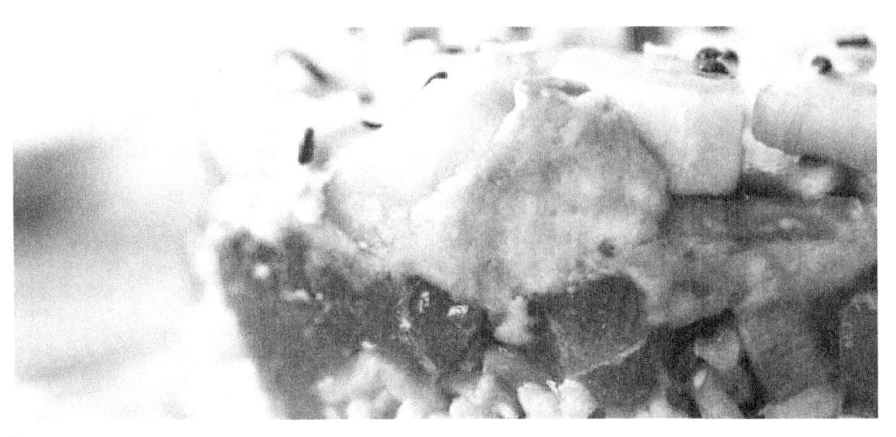

DIRECTION

1. Heat the oil in a medium (4 quart) pot over medium heat.
2. Add scallions and tarragon or basil and cook, stirring occasionally until scallions are soften, 4 minutes.
3. Add peas, stir for 1 minute. Add vegetable broth and bring mixture to a simmer and cook until peas are tender, 4 to 5 minutes.
4. Remove soup from heat and, working batches, use a blender to puree the soup with the mint until smooth.
5. Return the soup to a pot, stir in 2 tablespoons lemon juice and season with salt and pepper.
6. Keep soup warm until ready to serve.
7. Combine yogurt, lemon zest coriander and a pinch of salt.
8. Dollop soup servings with 2 1/4 teaspoons yogurt mixture just before serving.

LAYERED POTATO CUPS WITH SPRING HERBS AND LEEKS

5

NUTRITION:
Calories: 171kcal, Carbohydrates: 31g, Protein: 6g, Fat: 3.5g, Saturated Fat: 2.5g, Cholesterol: 6mg, Sodium: 409mg Fiber: 3g, Sugar: 3g

INGREDIENTS

- Olive oil spray
- 4 cups sliced leeks, sliced 1/4-inch thick (from about 3 to 4—white and lighter green parts only)
- 1 3/4 teaspoons kosher salt
- 3/4 teaspoons freshly ground black pepper
- 2 pounds Yukon Gold potatoes, peeled and sliced 1/16 inch thick
- 1 tablespoon chopped fresh thyme
- 1 tablespoon fresh chopped parsley, plus more for garnish
- 3 1/2 ounces garlic and herb cheese, such as Alouette Garlic Herb Spread Cheese, Goat Cheese or Boursin

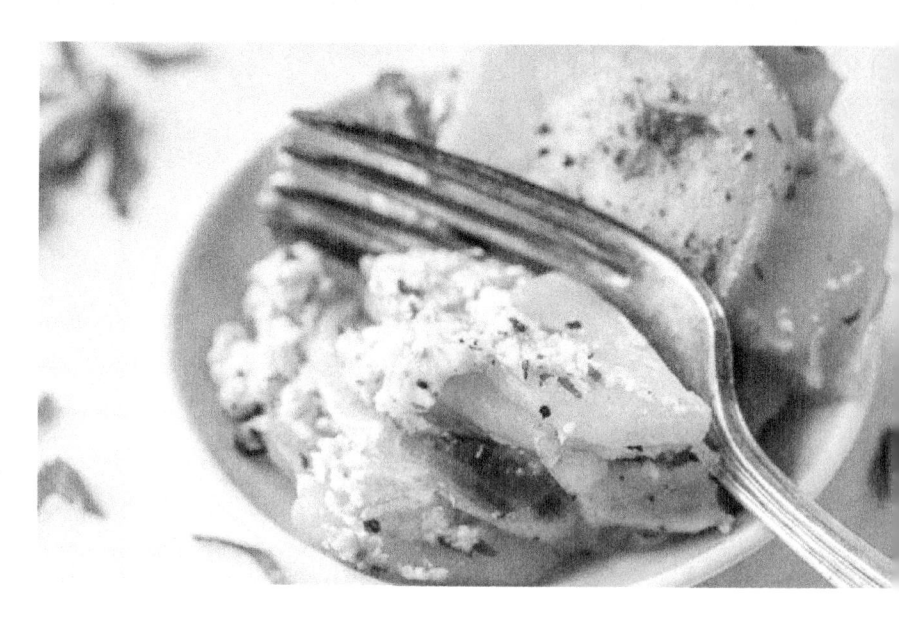

DIRECTION

1. Preheat over to 375°F.
2. Line a 12-cup muffin tin with foil liners. Lightly spray the liners with olive oil—use a brush if needed to ensure the sides are coated. Set aside.
3. Heat a large nonstick skillet over medium heat; spritz with the olive oil.
4. Add the leeks, 1/2 teaspoon salt and 1/4 teaspoon pepper and cook, stirring frequently, until leeks are soft, 4-5 minutes. Remove from heat and divide leeks into 12 equal portions, set aside.
5. Toss potato slices, thyme, 1 tablespoon parsley, remaining 1 1/4 teaspoon salt and remaining 1/2 teaspoon pepper together in a large bowl.
6. Evenly divide 1/3 of the potato slices and layer in the bottom of the prepared muffin cups.
7. Place about 1/2 of each portion of leeks (about 3/4 teaspoon), spreading out over the potato layer. Add another third of potatoes to the cups.
8. Evenly divide the goat cheese and press to spread out onto the potato layer (about a heaping teaspoon per muffin cup). Add the remaining leeks and then top each cup with the remaining potatoes.
9. Lightly spray the tops of each muffin cup with olive oil and cover the muffin tin with foil.
10. Bake for 30 minutes then remove foil and bake until potatoes are tender and easily pieces with knife, about 10 additional minutes.
11. Remove potato cups and invert and garnish with more fresh chopped parsley to serve.

SPANAKOPITA BAKED EGGS

3

NUTRITION:
Calories: 198kcal, Carbohydrates: 13.5g,
Protein: 15g, Fat: 11g, Saturated Fat: 5g,
Cholesterol: 205mg, Sodium: 703.5mg
Fiber: 6g, Sugar: 3g

INGREDIENTS

- 1-1/2 lbs frozen spinach, thawed [24 ounces]
- 1 tsp olive oil
- 1/2 medium yellow onion, thinly sliced [1 1/2 cups]
- 1 tsp kosher salt
- 1/2 cup chopped scallions , [3-5 scallions depending on the size]
- 1/2 cup chopped dill
- 3/4 cup crumbled feta
- Juice of 1 lemon
- Black pepper, to taste
- 4 large eggs

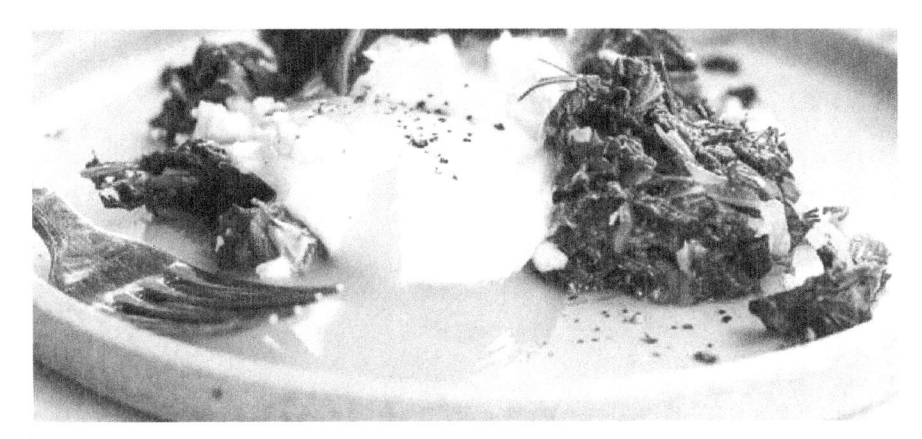

DIRECTION

1. Preheat the oven to 375°F degrees.
2. Squeeze most of the water out of the spinach, but you don't have to go crazy— a little water left is fine and will cook off in the oven.
3. Heat a large ovenproof skillet over medium-high heat. When hot, add 1 tsp olive oil, then add the onion and 1/2 tsp salt, and cook until tender and translucent, 3 to 5 minutes.
4. Add the scallions and cook, stirring constantly, until just starting to soften, about 1 minute.
5. Add the spinach, dill, 1/2 cup feta, lemon juice, remaining 1/2 tsp salt, and pepper and mix until everything is well-combined and heated through. Remove from the heat.
6. Make four wells in the top, crack an egg into each, and season each with a little salt and pepper.
7. Top spinach with remaining 1/4 cup Feta.
8. Carefully transfer the skillet to the middle rack and bake just until the egg whites are set, 8 to 13 minutes, to your desired liking.

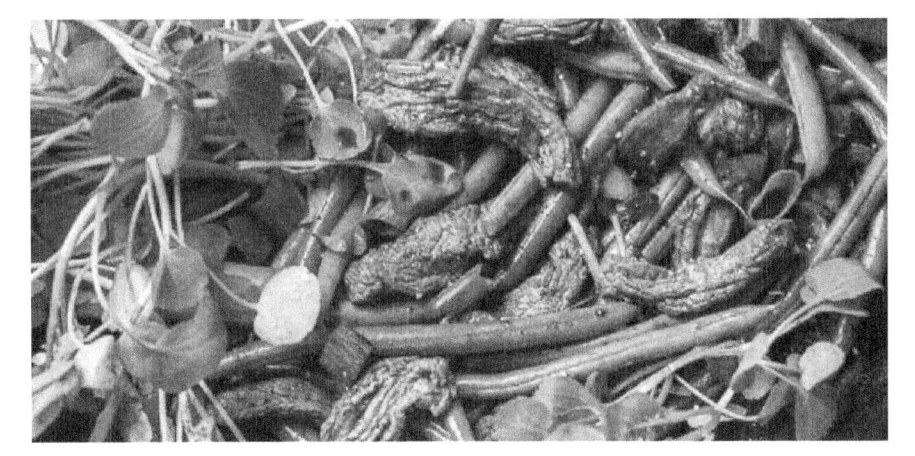

BEEF NEGIMAKI STIR FRY

5

NUTRITION:
Calories: 251kcal, Carbohydrates: 14g,
Protein: 28.5g, Fat: 7.5g, Saturated Fat: 3g,
Cholesterol: 78mg, Sodium: 1211mg
Fiber: 2.5g, Sugar: 9.5g

INGREDIENTS

- 1 pound flank steak
- Sea salt and freshly ground black pepper
- 1/4 cup sake or dry white wine, optional
- 1/4 cup gluten-free tamari or coconut aminos
- 2 tablespoons rice vinegar or white wine vinegar
- 1 tablespoon clover honey or pure maple syrup
- Coconut or avocado oil
- 8 ounces French green beans, cut in half
- 1 bunch scallions, green parts only, cut into 1-inch pieces
- 5 ounces watercress, about 4 cups packed

DIRECTION

1. Slice the steak as thinly as possible against the grain. Season generously with salt and pepper. Set aside.
2. In a small bowl, stir together the sake (if using), tamari, vinegar, and honey until dissolved.
3. Set a large wok or heavy-bottomed skillet over high heat. Add a thin layer of oil and arrange the steak in an even layer.
4. Brown the meat, flipping once, until there's a dark sear on both sides, about 3 minutes total. Transfer to a bowl.
5. Add the green beans and sauce to the pan. Simmer vigorously, stirring occasionally, until the sauce has reduced by half and the beans are al dente, about 3 minutes.
6. Return the beef to the pan along with the scallions and toss to coat in the sauce.
7. To serve, arrange the watercress on a platter and top with the beef stir-fry and sauce. Serve immediately alongside white rice, if you like.

SALMON, BEET, AND ARUGULA SALAD WITH PISTACHIOS AND POMEGRANATES

8

NUTRITION:
Calories: 437kcal, Carbohydrates: 18g, Protein: 33.5g, Fat: 26.5g, Saturated Fat: 8.3g, Cholesterol: 85mg, Sodium: 727.5mg, Fiber: 4.5g, Sugar: 12g

INGREDIENTS

- 1 Tbsp olive oil
- Olive oil spray
- 1 tsp white wine vinegar
- ½ tsp Dijon mustard
- ½ pound wild salmon, cut into 2 fillets
- Kosher salt
- 3 cups arugula
- 1 cup cooked beets, 6 to 8 oz, cut into small wedges
- 1 to 2 radishes, thinly sliced
- 2 oz fresh goat cheese, crumbled
- 2 Tbsp pistachios, toasted and chopped
- 2 Tbsp pomegranate seeds
- 1 Tbsp capers

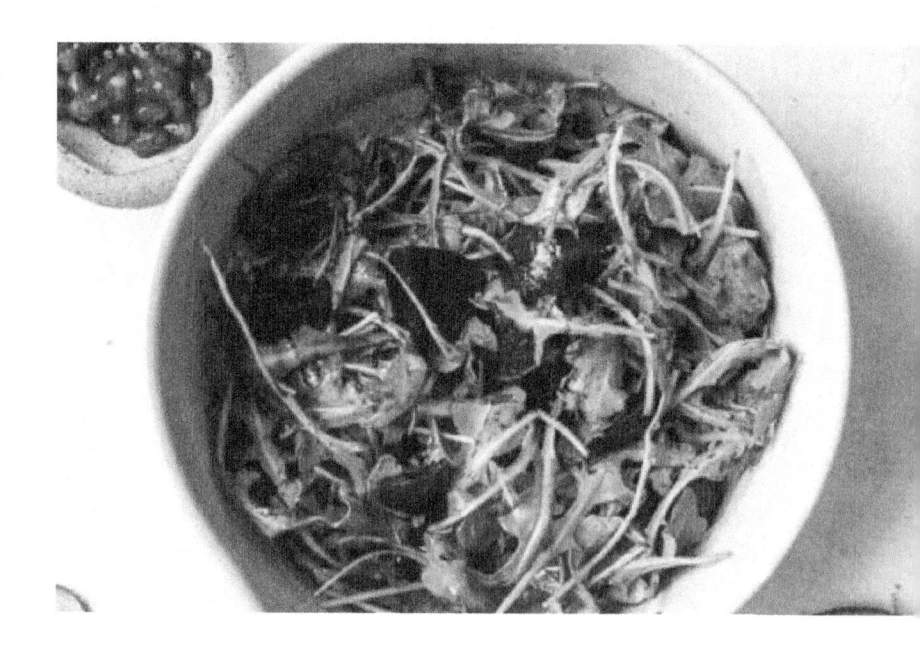

DIRECTION

1. Preheat the oven to 450°F. In a large bowl, combine 1 tbsp olive oil with the vinegar and mustard; set aside.
2. Set a heavy ovenproof skillet over medium-high heat and lightly spray or coat with olive oil.
3. Season the salmon on both sides with salt.
4. When the oil is very hot, add the salmon (skin side down if it's skin-on) and use your spatula to lightly press it down to help the skin sear.
5. Let cook undisturbed for 1 to 2 minutes, until the skin releases easily from the pan and the edges are opaque, then flip and transfer to the oven to finish cooking 2 to 4 minutes, depending on thickness and desired doneness. Set aside.
6. Add the arugula and beets to the bowl with the dressing and toss to coat; season to taste with salt.
7. Sprinkle in the radishes, goat cheese, pistachios, pomegranate seeds and capers.
8. Divide onto two plates and top with the salmon and capers.

SHEET PAN TERIYAKI SALMON AND VEGETABLES

8

NUTRITION:
Calories: 326kcal, Carbohydrates: 17g, Protein: 27g, Fat: 17g, Saturated Fat: 2.5g, Cholesterol: 62mg, Sodium: 758mg, Fiber: 4g, Sugar: 4g

INGREDIENTS

For vegetables:
- 2 cups bite-size broccoli florets
- 10 mini sweet rainbow peppers, seeded and halved
- 1 tablespoon sesame oil
- ¼ teaspoon kosher salt
- Freshly ground black pepper, to taste

For salmon:
- 2 (4-ounce) wild salmon filets
- 1 teaspoon sesame oil
- 1 garlic clove, grated
- ½ teaspoon grated ginger
- 2 tablespoons reduced sodium soy sauce, or gluten-free soy sauce
- 1 teaspoon unseasoned rice vinegar
- 1 teaspoon brown sugar

For garnish:
- ½ teaspoon toasted sesame seeds
- 1 large scallion, chopped

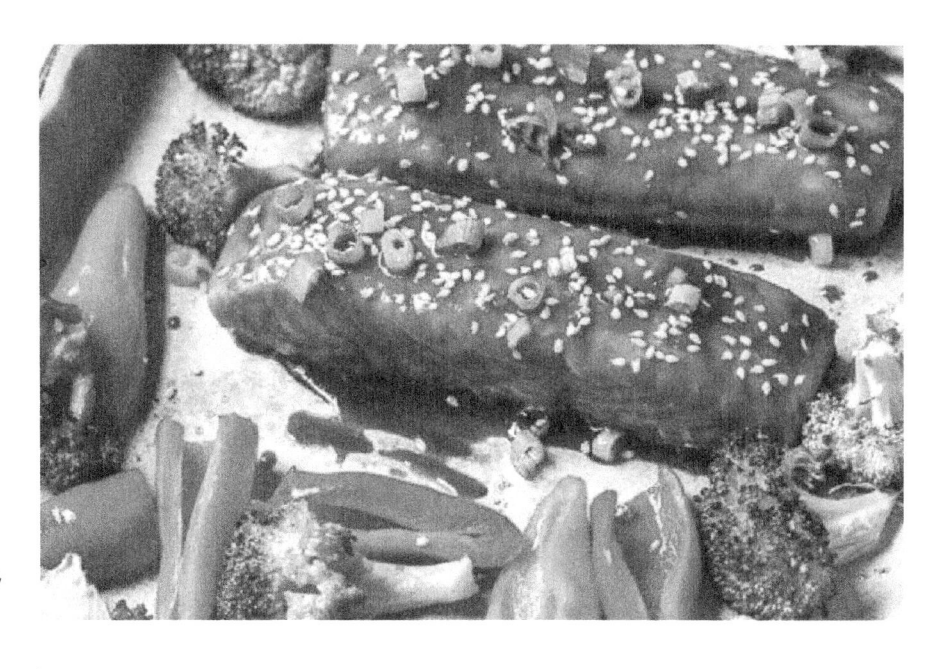

DIRECTION

1. Preheat oven to 400F degrees. Cover a large sheet pan with foil or parchment, lightly spray olive oil and set aside.
2. Meanwhile, combine sesame oil, garlic, ginger, soy sauce, vinegar and brown sugar in a small bowl and mix. Pour into a large ziplock bag and add salmon, marinate 10 minutes.
3. In a medium bowl, toss broccoli and peppers with 1 tablespoon sesame oil, ¼ teaspoon salt and pepper. Spread them evenly on prepared sheet pan and roast for 10 minutes.
4. Remove veggies from oven, toss, and move them over slightly to make room for the salmon. Place the salmon on the sheet pan, reserving the marinade and return to oven, roast an additional 7 to 8 minutes, or until salmon is just cooked through.
5. While salmon is cooking, heat a small skillet over low heat. Pour the remaining marinade and simmer stirring until the sauce has thickened slightly, about 1 to 1 1/2 minutes.
6. Brush sauce over salmon and sprinkle fillets with sesame seeds and scallions. Serve with veggies on the side.

CHEESY EGGPLANT GNOCCHI CAPRESE `11`

NUTRITION:
Calories: 436kcal, Carbohydrates: 66g, Protein: 15g, Fat: 11g, Saturated Fat: 5g, Cholesterol: 30mg, Sodium: 900mg, Fiber: 7g, Sugar: 5g

INGREDIENTS
- 16 oz package Delallo gnocchi
- 1 tbsp olive oil
- ½ large onion or 1 small onion, chopped
- 1 tsp kosher salt
- 1 lb eggplant, diced
- 2 cloves garlic, crushed
- 5- ounce container baby spinach
- 1 tbsp tomato paste
- 28- oz can San Marzano Style crushed tomatoes
- 6 leaves fresh basil
- 6 oz small mozzarella cheese balls

DIRECTION
1. Bring water to a boil, cook gnocchi according to package directions and drain.
2. Meanwhile, set a large nonstick skillet over medium heat and add the oil.
3. When the oil is warm, add the onion, eggplant and salt to the pan and saute for about 3 minutes, or until it begins to soften, then add the garlic and cook until fragrant, about 1 minute.
4. Gradually add the spinach, stirring until it wilts. Once it's all in the pan, saute for 1 to 2 minutes, or until it cooks down.
5. Push it to one side of the pan with your spoon and add the tomato paste, stirring until it smells lightly caramelized and toasty.
6. Pour in the can of tomatoes and decrease the heat to medium.
7. Cover the pan and cook for 5 to 6 minutes, or until the eggplant is tender.
8. Add the cooked gnocchi, place the mozzarella on top, cover the pan and cook 3 to 5 minutes, or until the mozzarella is melty.
9. Garnish with torn fresh basil and serve.

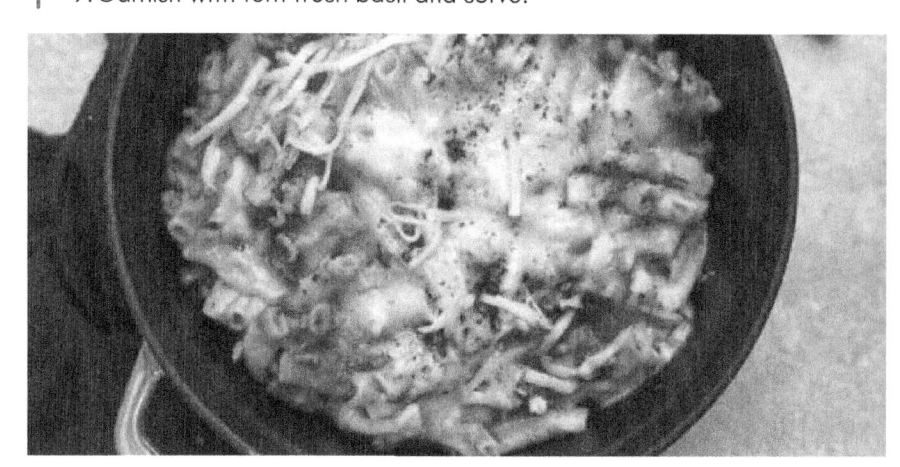

INSTANT POT BAKED ZITI
`10`

NUTRITION:
Calories: 452kcal, Carbohydrates: 64g, Protein: 24g, Fat: 12.5g, Saturated Fat: 5g, Cholesterol: 29.5mg, Sodium: 855.5mg Fiber: 10g, Sugar: 6.5g

INGREDIENTS
- 1 teaspoon olive oil
- 3 garlic cloves, smashed with the side of a knife
- 2 cups chopped baby spinach
- 2 cups water
- 3/4 teaspoon Kosher salt
- 10 ounces Delallo whole wheat pasta such as ziti or cavatappi, about 3 cups
- 2 cups homemade or jarred marinara sauce
- 1/2 cup part skim ricotta
- 1/4 cup grated Pecorino Romano
- 1 cup part-skim mozzarella cheese, grated

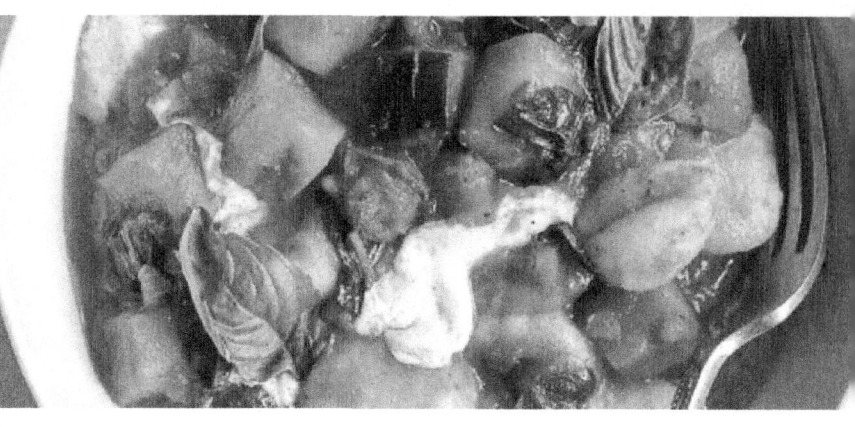

DIRECTION
1. Using the saute button, when hot add the oil and garlic; stir 1 minute, or until golden.
2. Add water and salt to the pot to deglaze, making sure the garlic is not stuck to the bottom of the pot.
3. Add spinach and pasta and stir.
4. Pour the marinara sauce evenly over the uncooked pasta, making sure it's covering all the pasta. Do not stir.
5. Cover and cook high pressure 7 minutes.
6. Quick release, then open the lid, stir the pasta, dollop in the ricotta, top with Pecorino and the mozzarella.
7. Cover the lid 3 to 4 minutes, until the cheese melts.

SHRIMP DUMPLING LETTUCE WRAPS OR RICE BOWLS

3

NUTRITION:
Calories: 201kcal, Carbohydrates: 9.5g, Protein: 25.5g, Fat: 6.5g, Saturated Fat: 1g, Cholesterol: 172.5mg, Sodium: 955.5mg, Fiber: 1.5g, Sugar: 3g

INGREDIENTS

Pickled carrots:
- ¼ cup plus 3 Tbsp rice vinegar, divided
- 2 tablespoons honey or sugar
- 1 cup shredded carrots

Shrimp and Sauce:
- ¼ cup plus 1 tbsp low sodium soy sauce
- 2 cloves garlic, minced
- 1 tablespoon sesame oil, plus 1 teaspoon more for cooking
- 2- in piece fresh ginger, peeled and divided
- 2 scallions
- 1 pound shrimp, peeled
- 1 teaspoon sriracha, plus more for serving
- 1 head Bibb or endive lettuce, leaves separated
- 3 cups brown rice, optional to make rice bowls

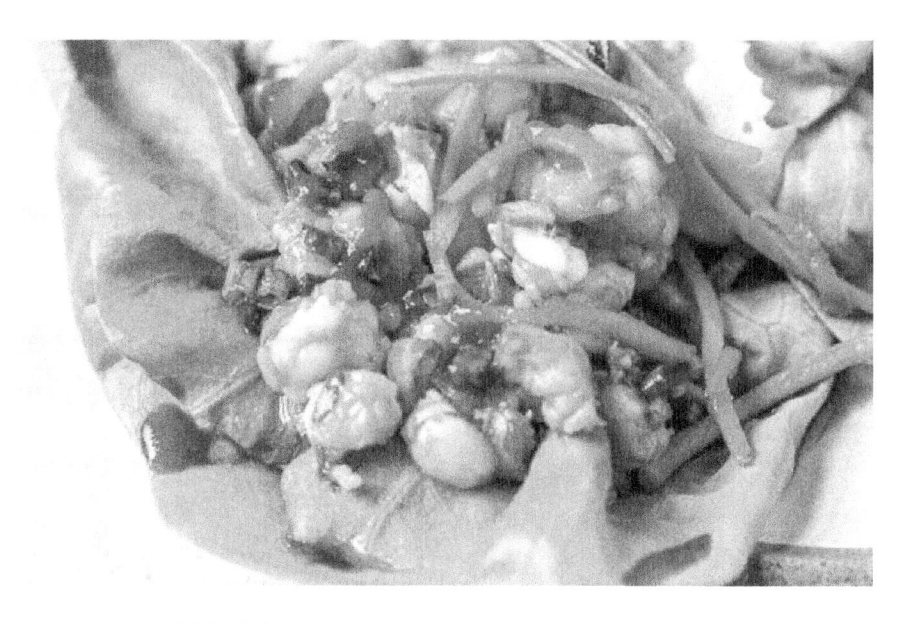

DIRECTION

To make the quick-pickled carrots
1. Combine ¼ cup rice vinegar with 2 Tbsp water and the honey or sugar. Add the carrots and stir to combine. Set aside.
2. To make the dumpling sauce:
3. Combine ¼ cup soy sauce with the remaining 3 Tbsp rice vinegar, garlic and sesame oil.
4. Thinly slice half the ginger (a 1-in piece) along with the dark green top of one scallion. Add to the dumpling sauce.

For the shrimp:
1. If you're using frozen shrimp, thaw it completely and drain as much water as possible, using a paper towel to pat it dry. Finely chop with a knife, until it's about the consistency of ground meat. Add to a large mixing bowl.
2. Mince the white and light green parts of the remaining scallions along with the remaining 1-in piece of ginger and add them to the bowl with the shrimp.
3. Season with the remaining 1 Tbsp soy sauce and (if using) the sriracha; stir until completely incorporated.
4. Set a large lidded skillet over medium heat with 1 tsp oil.
5. When the oil is hot, add the shrimp mixture and spread it in an even layer. Cook undisturbed for 1 to 2 minutes, then stir and cover to let the residual steam finish the cooking.
6. Drain the quick-pickled carrots.
7. To serve, wrap the filling in lettuce leaves and serve with pickled carrots, dumpling sauce, and (if using) more sriracha on the side.
8. If making rice bowls, omit the lettuce and serve over 3/4 cups cooked rice (not included in macros/points).

SHRIMP & ANDOUILLE SHEET PAN ROAST

6

NUTRITION:
Calories: 374kcal, Carbohydrates: 18g, Protein: 38g, Fat: 18g, Saturated Fat: 3.5g, Cholesterol: 189mg, Sodium: 1050.5mg Fiber: 6.5g, Sugar: 6.5g

INGREDIENTS

- ¾ pound large shrimp, peeled
- 2 Tbsp olive oil, divided
- 1 ½ tsp Creole seasoning, divided
- 1 small head broccoli
- 5 oz Baby Bella mushrooms
- 2 to 3 stalks celery
- 1 red bell pepper, sliced
- ½ large red onion, sliced
- ¾ pound smoked sausage, preferably andouille, sliced
- ½ tsp garlic powder
- ¼ tsp cayenne pepper
- 1 lemon, for serving
- Steamed rice, optional for serving

DIRECTION

1. Preheat the oven to 400F.
2. If you're using frozen shrimp, thaw it completely and drain as much water as possible, using a paper towel to pat it dry.
3. Toss to coat with 1 Tbsp olive oil and ½ tsp Creole seasoning; set aside.
4. Cut the broccoli into florets, halve the mushroom caps (quarter the larger ones), and cut the celery into approximately 2-inch pieces.
5. Add them to a large rimmed baking sheet with the sliced bell pepper, onion, and smoked sausage.
6. Drizzle 1 Tbsp olive oil over the sheet pan and season with 1 tsp Creole seasoning, the garlic powder, and the cayenne. Toss to coat, then spread in an even layer.
7. Roast for 15 to 20 minutes, or until the vegetables are tender and the onions are just starting to brown around the edges.
8. Add the shrimp and roast for another 5 to 10 minutes, or until it's firm, opaque, and cooked through.
9. To serve, zest the lemon and squeeze its juice over the roast.
10. Serve with steamed rice if you'd like.

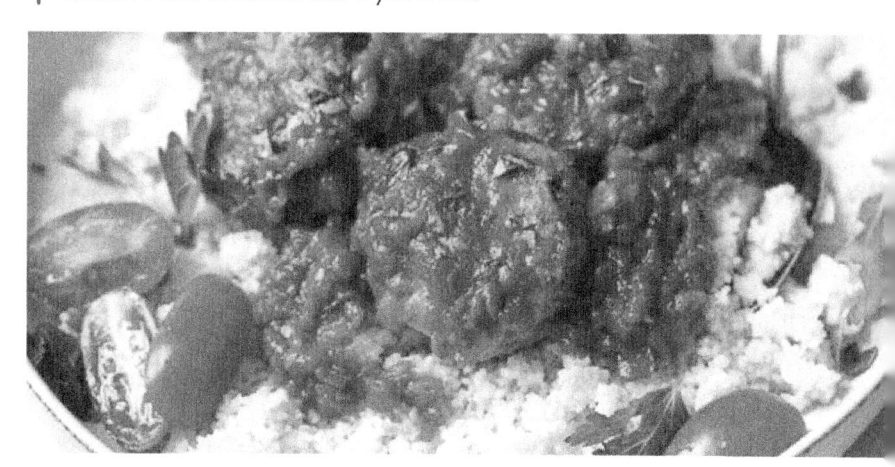

HARISSA CHICKEN MEATBALLS

8

NUTRITION:
Calories: 290kcal, Carbohydrates: 12.5g, Protein: 22g, Fat: 20.5g, Saturated Fat: 3g, Cholesterol: 142.5mg, Sodium: 1520mg Fiber: 11g, Sugar: 11g

INGREDIENTS

- 1 pound ground chicken
- 1 teaspoon kosher salt
- 1/2 teaspoon smoked paprika
- 1/2 cup frozen riced cauliflower
- 1/4 cup chopped onion
- 1/4 cup packed chopped parsley
- 3 large peeled garlic cloves, minced
- 1 large egg
- Olive-oil cooking spray
- 2 jars, 10 oz each prepared mild harissa sauce

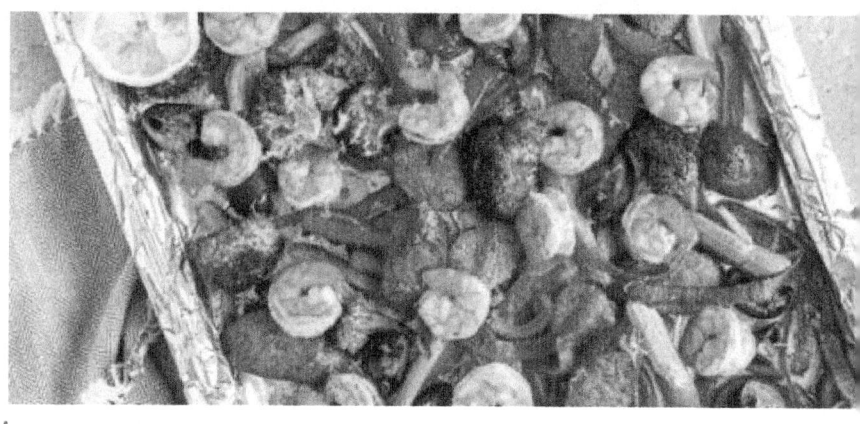

DIRECTION

1. Place chicken in a large mixing bowl, break-up slightly. Sprinkle with 1 teaspoon salt and smoked paprika.
2. Add frozen cauliflower, parsley, onion, garlic, and egg and mix just until ingredients are combined. Avoid over-mixing. Divide chicken mixture into 16 portions (about 1 1/4 ounce each); gently shape into balls.
3. Heat a heavy-duty non-stick large skillet (with tall sides) over medium-high heat.
4. Spray with olive oil cooking spray, add meatballs and cook, turning occasionally to brown on all sides, about 6 minutes.
5. Pour in harissa and allow mixture to reach a simmer, reduce heat to medium-low and continue to simmer for 20 to 25 minutes.

HOUSE SPECIAL FRIED RICE

7

NUTRITION:
Calories: 432kcal, Carbohydrates: 40.5g,
Protein: 35g, Fat: 14g, Saturated Fat: 3g,
Cholesterol: 200mg, Sodium: 598.5mg
Fiber: 4g, Sugar: 3g

INGREDIENTS

- 8 ounces peeled and deveined shrimp, chopped
- 6 ounces thin sliced chicken breast cutlet, sliced into 1/4 inch thin strips
- 6 ounces thin sliced sirloin steak, sliced into 1/4 inch thin strips
- 1/4 teaspoon kosher salt
- 2 1/2 teaspoons vegetable or canola oil, divided
- 1 tablespoon chopped fresh ginger
- 2 garlic cloves, chopped
- 4 medium scallions, thinly sliced, whites and greens separated
- 2 cups frozen riced cauliflower
- 3 cups cooked cold leftover brown rice, preferably short-grain
- 2 large eggs, beaten
- 2 tablespoons soy sauce, or gluten-free Tamari
- 1 tablespoon rice vinegar
- 1 1/2 teaspoons toasted sesame oil
- Sriracha or Chile-garlic sauce, optional for serving

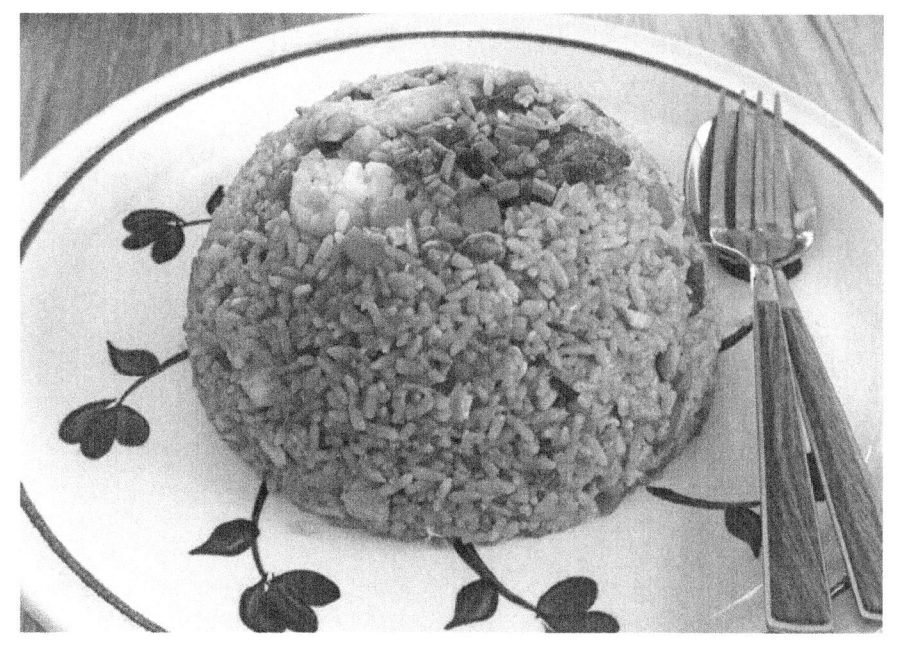

DIRECTION

1. The easiest way to get the chicken and steak sliced into thin strips is to roll the thin piece of meat, then slice it.
2. Season the shrimp, chicken and steak with salt.
3. Heat a large nonstick wok or deep skillet over medium-high heat. When hot spritz with oil and add the steak, cook about 2 to 3 minutes turning halfway then set aside on a plate.
4. Add the chicken, cook 2 to 3 minutes, stirring and set aside with the beef.
5. Add the shrimp and cook 2 to 3 minutes, stirring. Set aside with the other meat.
6. Heat 1 teaspoon of the oil in a large nonstick wok or deep skillet over medium- high.
7. Add ginger, garlic and the scallion whites and cook, stirring, until fragrant, about 1 minute. Add the cauliflower and cook, stirring occasionally, until heated, 3 to 4 minutes. Push to one side.
8. Add the remaining 1/2 tablespoon oil and swirl around the skillet to evenly transfer, add the cooked rice in an even layer.
9. Cook, without stirring, 2 to 3 minutes, or until the bottom becomes slightly crispy.
10. Continue to cook, stirring occasionally, 1 to 2 minutes, or until combined.
11. With a spoon or spatula, push the rice to one side of the wok or skillet. Crack the eggs onto the other side.
12. Cook, constantly stirring the egg, 30 to 60 seconds or until cooked through. Mix the rice and egg to thoroughly combine.
13. Return the reserved shrimp, steak and chicken and scallion greens to the skillet and toss until warmed.
14. Stir in the soy sauce, rice vinegar and sesame oil.
15. Serve immediately. Serve with sriracha sauce, if desired.

SHRIMP PHO WITH VEGETABLES

5

NUTRITION:
Calories: 233kcal, Carbohydrates: 19.5g, Protein: 30.5g, Fat: 2.5g, Saturated Fat: 0.5g, Cholesterol: 172.5mg, Sodium: 1548.5mg, Fiber: 3.5g, Sugar: 4g

INGREDIENTS

- 1 pound large shrimp
- 1 ½ quarts vegetable or chicken broth
- 1 Tbsp fish sauce
- 1 Tbsp soy sauce
- 1 cinnamon stick
- 1 star anise pod
- 1- in piece ginger, sliced
- 8 oz white mushrooms, halved
- 1 bunch cilantro
- Salt to taste
- 6 ounces thin rice noodles
- 3 cups cauliflower or broccoli, from 1 small head
- Garnish: Thinly sliced jalapeno, lime wedges,, mung bean sprouts, fresh mint, Thai basil, sliced scallions, sriracha, and/or hoisin sauce

DIRECTION

1. If you're using frozen shrimp, thaw it completely and drain as much water as possible, using a paper towel to pat it dry.
2. If you're using fresh, shell-on shrimp, peel it and reserve the shells for the stock.
3. Add the broth, fish sauce, soy sauce, cinnamon stick, star anise pod, sliced ginger, and (if applicable) shrimp shells to a medium saucepan and bring to a simmer. Chop the leafy tops from the bunch of cilantro. Add all the stems to the saucepan.
4. Cook for 20 to 25 minutes, or until very fragrant, then use a slotted spoon to remove and discard the solids. Keep at a gentle simmer.
5. Meanwhile, just before the broth is ready fill a wide skillet with water and bring to a boil over high heat, then remove from heat and add the rice noodles.
6. Let soak for 3 to 5 minutes, or according to package instructions. Drain and set aside. Add the mushrooms and cauliflower florets to the broth and cook for 4 to 5 minutes, or until tender but still crisp.
7. Add the shrimp and cook for 1 to 2 minutes, until firm, opaque, and pink.

To serve:
1. Divide the rice noodles to each bowl first, then use a slotted spoon to distribute the shrimp and veggies, about 1 1/4 cup each.
2. Ladle 1 cup broth over the top. Serve with lime wedges and sriracha.

DRUNKEN SHRIMP

3

NUTRITION:
Calories: 175kcal, Carbohydrates: 2g, Protein: 22.5g, Fat: 10g, Saturated Fat: 2g, Cholesterol: 185mg, Sodium: 861mg Fiber: 0.3g, Sugar: 0.1g

INGREDIENTS

- 2 tsp extra virgin olive oil
- 2 tsp unsalted butter
- 1 tsp anchovy paste
- 1 lb peeled and deveined large or jumbo shrimp
- 6 garlic cloves, chopped
- 1 tsp crushed red pepper flakes
- fresh pepper to taste
- 1/4 cup of white wine
- 1 cup clam juice
- 2 tablespoons of capers, rinsed
- generous handful of chopped parsley

DIRECTION

1. Heat olive oil and butter in a skillet over medium heat. Add garlic, pepper flakes, and sauté 1 to 2 minutes, until golden.
2. Add wine, clam juice, lemon juice, capers, anchovy paste, parsley, salt and pepper, and stir. Bring to a boil and cook for another 2-3 minutes.
3. Add the shrimp and cook, stirring for 2-3 minutes, until opaque. Do not overcook the shrimp or it will become tough and chewy.
4. Serve shrimp with liquid in a bowl and some crusty bread on the side to soak up the juice.

COLOMBIAN STEAK WITH ONIONS AND TOMATOES | 4

NUTRITION:
Calories: 188kcal, Carbohydrates: 3g, Protein: 25.2g, Fat: 7.2g, Saturated Fat: 0.5g, Sodium: 49mg, Fiber: 0.7g

INGREDIENTS

- 1-1/2 lbs sirloin tip steak, sliced very thin
- kosher salt to taste
- 1/2 teaspoon garlic powder
- 1/2 teaspoon cumin
- 4 tsp olive oil
- 1 medium onion, sliced thin or chopped
- 1 very large tomato or 2 medium tomatoes, sliced thin or chopped
- cooked rice and fried eggs, optional for serving

DIRECTION

1. Season steak with 1 teaspoon salt and garlic powder.
2. Heat a large frying pan until VERY HOT.
3. Add 2 tsp of oil then half of the steak and cook less than a minute on each side until browned.
4. Set steak aside, add another teaspoon of oil and cook remaining steak. Set aside.
5. Reduce heat to medium, add another teaspoon of oil and add the onions.
6. Cook 2 minutes, until soft then add the tomatoes.
7. Season with more salt, to taste, about 1/4 to 1/2 teaspoon. Add black pepper and cumin and reduce heat to medium-low.
8. Add 1/4 cup of water and simmer a few minutes to create a sauce, add more water if needed and taste adjust seasoning as needed.
9. Return the steak to the pan along with the drippings, combine well and remove from heat.
10. Serve over rice or veggie rice for a low carb option with a sunny-side up egg on top.

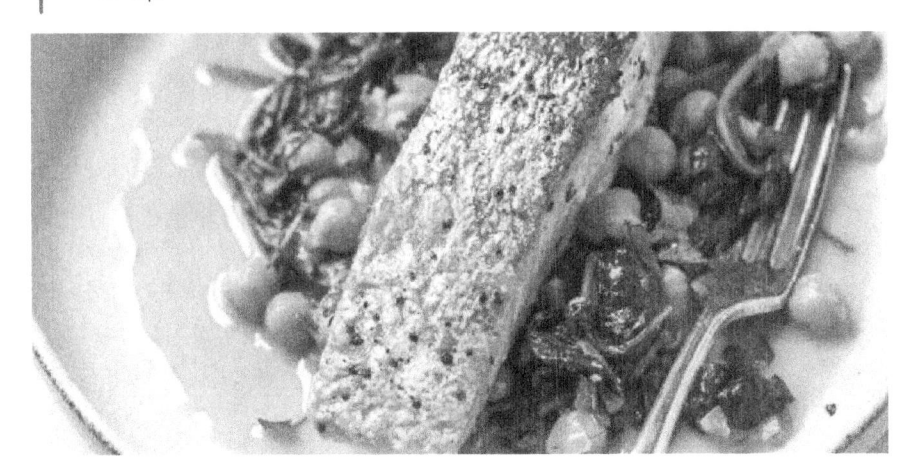

SALMON COCONUT CURRY WITH SPINACH AND CHICKPEAS | 4

NUTRITION:
Calories: 290kcal, Carbohydrates: 12.5g, Protein: 22g, Fat: 20.5g, Saturated Fat: 3g, Cholesterol: 142.5mg, Sodium: 1520mg, Fiber: 11g, Sugar: 11g

INGREDIENTS

- 1/2 teaspoon kosher salt, plus more to taste
- 1/4 teaspoon freshly ground black pepper
- 4 6-ounce skin-on salmon filets
- 2 teaspoons olive oil, divided
- 1 small onion, diced (about 1 small)
- 3 peeled garlic cloves, grated
- 1 2-inch piece peeled ginger, grated
- 1 large Fresno chili, finely diced
- 1 15-oz can chickpeas, rinsed and drained
- 1 1/2 teaspoons Madras curry powder
- 1 14-ounce can light coconut milk
- 5 ounces baby spinach

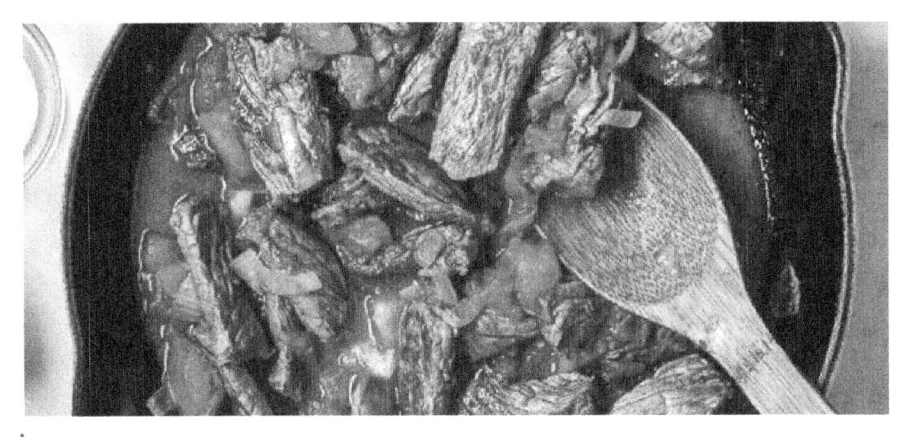

DIRECTION

1. Season both sides of salmon with 1/2 teaspoon salt and 1/4 teaspoon black pepper. Set aside on a plate.
2. Heat 1 teaspoon oil in a large skillet over medium-high heat. Spray with oil to fully coat the bottom of the pan.
3. Add salmon to the pan, skin-side down, and cook without disturbing until skin is crispy, 5 to 6 minutes. Return to the plate (skin-side up) and set aside.
4. Add remaining teaspoon of oil, then add onions, garlic, ginger, and Fresno chili pepper; cook, stirring, for 2 minutes.
5. Add chickpeas and curry powder and continue to cook, stirring, for 2 minutes more. Reduce heat to medium-low, add coconut milk, stirring, to release any browned bits stuck to the pan.
6. Stir in spinach and 1/2 teaspoon salt. Cover the pan and cook 2 minutes until spinach wilts.
7. Add the salmon, skin-side-up, and cook until fish is done, about 5 to 6 minutes.

SPINACH TOMATO FETA STUFFED CHICKEN BREAST

6

NUTRITION:
Calories: 407kcal, Carbohydrates: 7g, Protein: 44.5g, Fat: 22g, Saturated Fat: 6.5g, Cholesterol: 148mg, Sodium: 830mg Fiber: 1.5g, Sugar: 3.5g

INGREDIENTS

- 4 organic boneless, skinless chicken breasts, about 6 oz each
- 3/4 tsp kosher salt
- 3/4 tsp paprika
- 1/2 tsp garlic powder

Filling:

- 1 cup baby spinach, chopped
- 2/3 cup sundried tomatoes in oil, drained and chopped
- 2/3 cups crumbled feta cheese
- 1 medium shallot, chopped
- 1 large garlic clove, minced
- 1/4 cup chopped fresh basil
- 2 tablespoons plain or gluten-free panko
- 1 tablespoon chopped fresh oregano
- 1 tablespoon grated Parmesan cheese
- 1/4 teaspoon kosher salt
- 1 tablespoon olive oil, divided

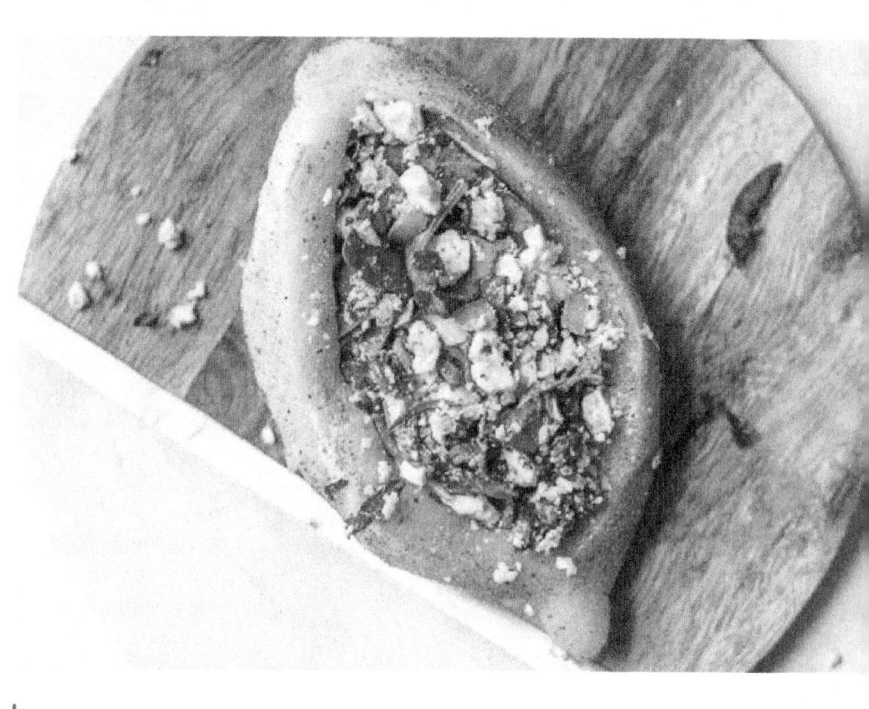

DIRECTION

1. Preheat oven to 425°F.
2. Use a sharp knife to slice a pocket into the sides of each chicken breast. Make sure you don't cut all the way through, just enough to create a place for the spinach mixture to go.
3. Season both sides of each chicken breast with 3/4 teaspoon salt, paprika and garlic powder. Set aside.
4. In a medium bowl combine the sun dried tomatoes, spinach, feta cheese, shallots, garlic, basil, panko, oregano, parmesan cheese, salt and 1/2 tablespoon olive oil.
5. Mix well and set aside.
6. Divide spinach mixture between the chicken breasts and stuff into each, about 3/4 cup each. If needed, you can use toothpicks to close chicken breast.
7. Heat a large, oven-safe or cast iron skillet over medium heat.
8. Add the remaining oil and once hot, sear the chicken breasts on each side for about 2 to 3 minutes, until browned.
9. Transfer skillet to oven and finish cooking 12 to 15 minutes, until chicken reaches 165°F.
10. Remove from oven and tent with foil for 5 minutes before eating.
11. Remove toothpicks and eat right away.

SHEET PAN SHRIMP OREGANATA

3

NUTRITION:
Calories: 333kcal, Carbohydrates: 6g, Protein: 47.5g, Fat: 11.5g, Saturated Fat: 2g, Cholesterol: 346mg, Sodium: 442mg Fiber: 0.5g, Sugar: 0.5g

INGREDIENTS

- Reynolds Wrap Non-Stick Foil
- 2 pounds extra jumbo or collosal shrimp, 8 - 12 per pound (about 20)
- 2 tablespoons dry white wine
- 1/4 teaspoon kosher salt
- 1/4 teaspoon crushed red pepper flakes
- 3 tablespoons whole wheat bread crumbs
- 2 tablespoons fresh minced parsley
- 1 1/2 tablespoons grated Pecorino Romano cheese
- 2 cloves garlic, minced
- 1/2 teaspoon dried oregano
- 1 teaspoon lemon zest
- 2 tablespoon extra virgin olive oil
- fresh lemon wedges, for serving

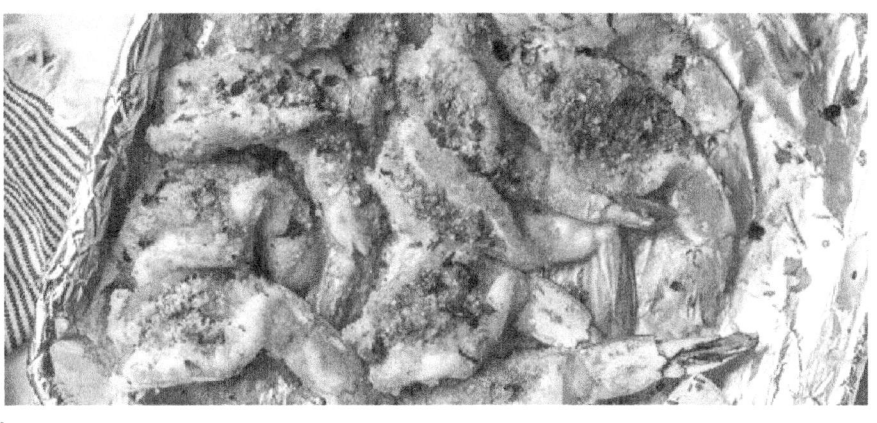

DIRECTION

1. Preheat the oven to 450°F, line a sheet pan with Reynolds Wrap Non-Stick Foil with the dull side facing up (the non-stick side).
2. Peel, devein, and butterfly the shrimp open, leaving the tails on.
3. Place the shrimp in a large bowl and toss gently with wine, salt, and crushed red pepper flakes. Set aside.
4. In a mixing bowl combine the breadcrumbs, parsley, pecorino cheese, garlic, oregano and lemon zest.
5. Add the shrimp to the sheet pan and arrange in a single layer cut side up.
6. Spoon the breadcrumb mixture over each shrimp and drizzle the top with extra virgin olive oil.
7. Bake until the shrimp are cooked through, about 8 to 10 minutes.
8. Broil on high for 2 minutes until the breadcrumbs are golden brown.
9. Serve with a squeeze of fresh lemon juice.

SLOW COOKER BUTTERNUT PEAR SOUP

2

NUTRITION:
Calories: 132kcal, Carbohydrates: 25.5g, Protein: 3g, Fat: 3g, Saturated Fat: 2.5g, Sodium: 275mg, Fiber: 6g, Sugar: 10g

INGREDIENTS

- 2 lbs butternut squash, halved, seeds removed (1 medium)
- 2 small ripe pears, peeled, cored and diced
- 2 large shallot, quartered
- 1 tablespoon fresh grated ginger
- 2 1/4 cup chicken or vegetable broth, or 1-1/2 tbsp Better Bouillon w/water
- 1/2 cup coconut milk, plus more optional for garnish
- pinch nutmeg
- 1/4 teaspoon kosher salt

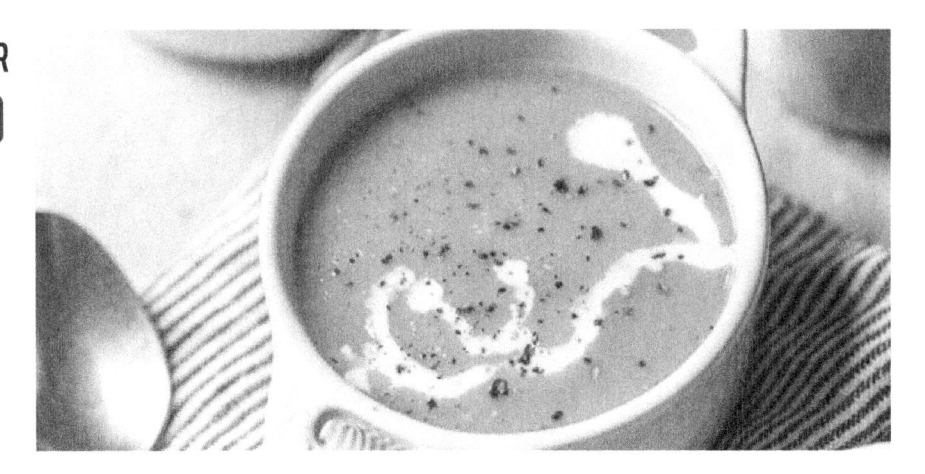

DIRECTION

1. Place the squash, pears, shallots, ginger and broth in the slow cooker.
2. Cook on low for 8 hours or high 4 hours, until soft and cooked through, a knife should easily be inserted.
3. Remove squash from skin and discard the peel.
4. Stir in coconut milk and nutmeg.
5. Blend in a blender or using an immersion blender until smooth.
6. Season with 1/4 teaspoon salt and black pepper and garnish with more coconut milk, if desired.

FRENCHED RACK OF LAMB

6

NUTRITION:
Calories: 335kcal, Carbohydrates: 0.5g, Protein: 46.7g, Fat: 16g, Saturated Fat: 7g, Cholesterol: 140mg, Sodium: 352.5mg Sugar: 0.5g

INGREDIENTS

- 4 cloves garlic, crushed
- 1 teaspoon chopped fresh rosemary leaves
- 2 racks of lamb, frenched (2 pounds each, 8 ribs each)
- 1/4 lemon
- 1 1/2 teaspoons kosher salt and freshly ground pepper, to taste

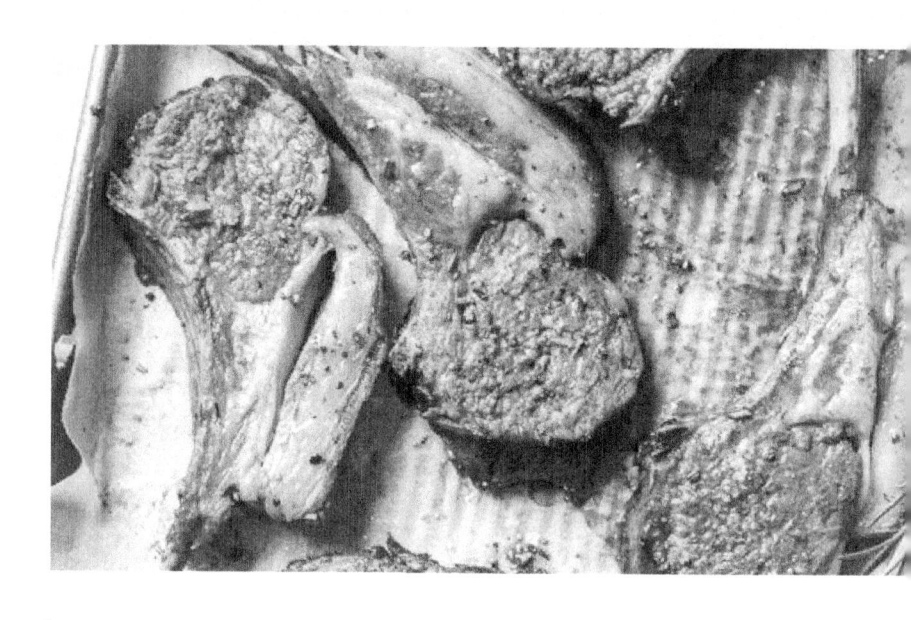

DIRECTION

1. Season the lamb racks with lemon juice and season with salt and pepper on both sides.
2. Rub the garlic all over them and sprinkle with rosemary.
3. Set the racks fat side up on a large rimmed baking sheet lined with foil if desired and let stand for 1 hour.
4. Preheat the oven to 450°F.
5. Roast the lamb in the upper third of the oven for about 25 minutes for medium-rare meat, or until a thermometer reaches 130F (or longer if you like your cooked medium or medium-well). Simply insert the tip of the thermometer through the side of the chops and into the thickest part of the meat, careful not to touch the bone (which is hotter than the meat that surrounds it).
6. When that spot reaches 130°F, it's finished. The temperature will continue to rise an additional 5 degrees as the lamb rests.
7. Transfer the lamb racks to a carving board and let them rest, tented with foil for 10 minutes.
8. Carve the lamb in between the rib bones and transfer to plates.
9. Serve right away. Trim fat before eating.

CHICKEN PARMESAN ROLLS

6

NUTRITION:
Calories: 259kcal, Carbohydrates: 28g,
Protein: 27.5g, Fat: 4.5g, Saturated Fat: 1.5g,
Cholesterol: 55.5mg, Sodium: 574mg
Fiber: 1.5g, Sugar: 2.5g

INGREDIENTS

For the dough:
- 1 cup all purpose or white whole wheat flour, plus more for dusting (5 oz)
- 1 1/2 teaspoons baking powder
- 1/2 teaspoon kosher salt
- 1 cup Stonyfield non-fat Greek yogurt, not regular, drained if there's any liquid

For the filling:
- 8 ounces organic grilled chicken breast, sliced (abut 2 cups)
- 1/2 cup marinara sauce
- 3/4 cup shredded part-skim mozzarella cheese
- For the egg wash:
- 1 large egg
- sesame seeds

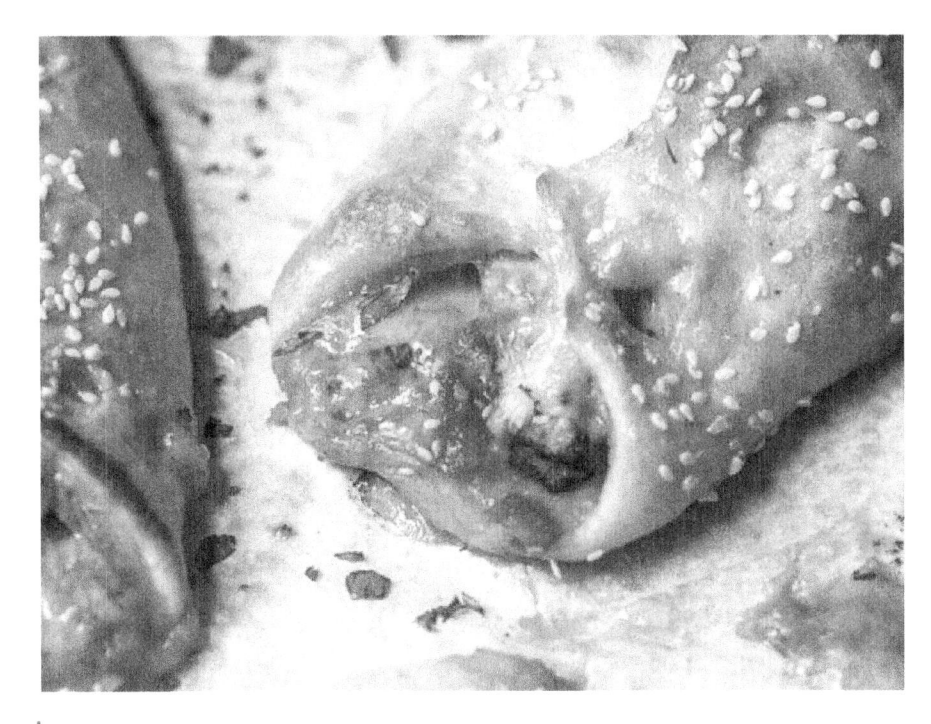

DIRECTION

1. In a medium bowl combine the flour, baking powder and salt and whisk well.
2. Add the yogurt and mix with a fork or spatula until well combined, it will look like small crumbles.
3. Lightly dust flour on a work surface and remove dough from the bowl, knead the dough a few times until smooth, not lumps. The dough will be tacky, but not sticky, about 20 turns (it should not leave dough on your hand when you pull away).
4. Preheat the oven 425F. Line a sheet pan with a silicone mat.

Assemble the rolls:

1. Divide into 4 equal balls, about 3-3/8 ounces each.
2. Lightly sprinkle a work surface and rolling pin with flour and roll the dough out into thin rounds, 7 inches in diameter.
3. Spread 1 tablespoon of marinara down the center of the circle in a strip, top with 1/2 cup of the chicken (2 oz) 1 tablespoon more marinara sauce and 3 tablespoons of cheese.
4. Fold the right side of the dough over the top of the chicken then repeat with the left side.
5. Brush the top with egg wash and sprinkle with sesame seeds.
6. Bake until golden, 20 minutes. Serve hot.

TURKEY POT PIE WITH STUFFING CRUST

4

NUTRITION:
Calories: 390kcal, Carbohydrates: 29.5g, Protein: 49.5g, Fat: 7.5g, Saturated Fat: 2g, Cholesterol: 140.5mg, Sodium: 760.5mg, Fiber: 4g, Sugar: 2g

INGREDIENTS

- 5 cups cooked diced turkey breast, (about 2+1/2 pounds)
- 1 tablespoon olive oil
- 2 large shallots, chopped (3/4 cup)
- 1/4 cup chopped fresh parsley
- 2 tablespoons chopped fresh thyme
- 2 tablespoons chopped fresh sage
- 3 celery stalks, chopped
- 8 ounce package frozen mixed vegetables
- 3 cups turkey or chicken broth
- 1/2 teaspoon kosher salt
- 1/8 teaspoon black pepper
- 1/4 cup cornstarch

For the Stuffing Crust:

- 10 ounces whole wheat french bread, cut into small cubes
- 1 tablespoon butter
- 1 medium onion, minced
- 2 large stalks celery, minced
- 8 fresh sage leaves, minced
- 1/2 cup chopped parsley
- 1 teaspoon Bell's turkey seasoning
- 1/4 teaspoon kosher salt and fresh pepper, to taste
- 1 large egg, beaten
- 1 1/2 cups chicken broth

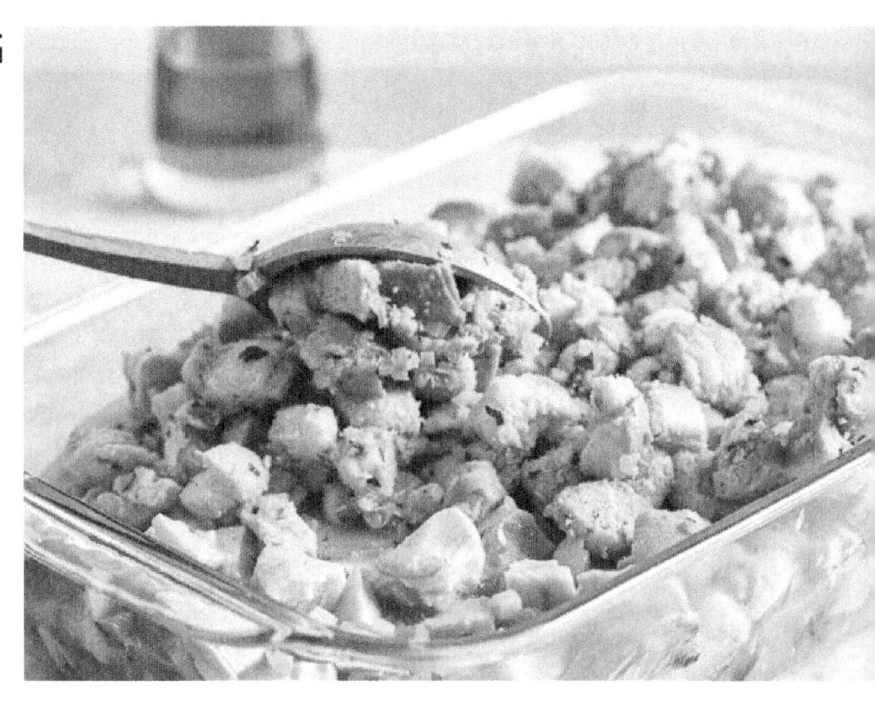

DIRECTION

For the stuffing crust:

1. Stale cubed bread works best here, you can cut the bread the night before and let it sit to harden.
2. If your bread is fresh, preheat the oven and bake the bread cubes on 2 baking sheets at 250°F for about 30 minutes, stirring half way until the bread is completely firm.
3. In a large, deep nonstick skillet over medium heat and add the butter; when melted add onions, celery, parsley, sage, Bell's turkey seasoning, 1/4 teaspoon salt and pepper and saute on medium low until soft, about 5-10 minutes.
4. Remove from heat and let cool a few minutes then transfer to a large bowl and add the toasted bread. Combine egg and broth in a bowl and whisk, add to the stuffing and mix to combine.

For the filling:

1. Preheat oven to 425F.
2. Wipe the skillet and add oil over medium heat. Add the shallots, parsley, thyme and sage and cook until almost soft about 2 to 3 minutes.
3. Add the celery and cook until the vegetables are soft, about 3 to 5 minutes.
4. Add the frozen mixed vegetables, turkey, 2 cups turkey broth, 1/2 teaspoon salt and black pepper and bring to a boil. Stir and simmer over medium-low heat 10 minutes, stirring until the flavors meld.
5. Meanwhile combine 1 cup turkey broth with the corn starch and mix well to dissolve.
6. Add to the turkey and cook over medium-low heat, stirring until thickened, about 4 to 6 minutes. Remove from heat and transfer to an oven safe, deep 9 x 13-inch baking dish.
7. Place the stuffing over the turkey filling. Bake 30 to 45 minutes, or until the crust is golden and the filling is hot and bubbling.

MEATLOAF AND BROWN GRAVY

7

NUTRITION:
Calories: 278kcal, Carbohydrates: 12g, Protein: 26.5g, Fat: 13.5g, Saturated Fat: 4g, Cholesterol: 125mg, Sodium: 688.5mg Fiber: 1.5g, Sugar: 2g

INGREDIENTS

- 1 tablespoon extra virgin olive oil
- 1 large yellow onion, chopped fine
- 2 medium celery stalks, minced fine
- 1 1/2 pounds 90% lean ground beef
- 1 1/2 pounds 93% lean ground turkey
- 1 tablespoon chopped parsley, plus more for garnish
- 1 tablespoon chopped fresh thyme leaves
- 3 large eggs, lightly beaten
- 1/2 cup fat free milk
- 4 teaspoons kosher salt
- 1 3/4 cups raw quick oats
- Beef Gravy: (makes 3 cups)
- 1/4 cup all purpose or gluten-free flour
- 3 cups salted beef broth or stock
- 1 thyme sprig
- fresh black pepper, to taste

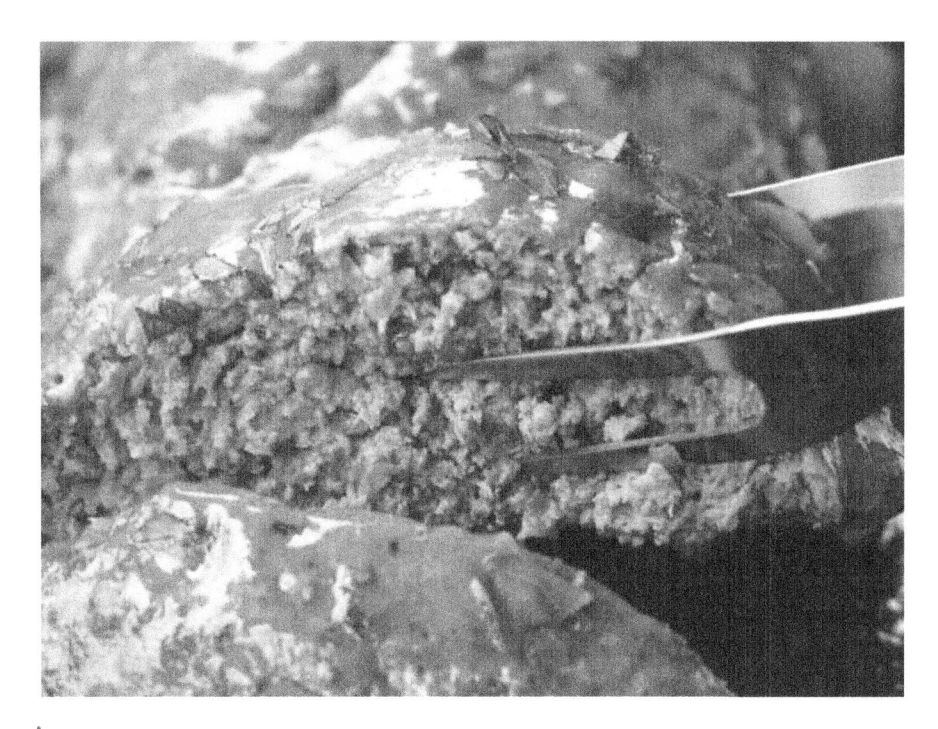

DIRECTION

1. Preheat the oven to 350F degrees. Place a piece of parchment paper or foil on a sheet pan.
2. Heat the olive oil in a large skillet over medium heat. Add the onion and celery and cook stirring occasionally, until the vegetables are soft, about 7 minutes.
3. Set aside to cool slightly.
4. In a large bowl combine the beef, turkey, parsley, thyme, eggs, milk, salt, and pepper.
5. Add the onion mixture and the oats and combine with clean hands until mixed well.
6. Form into 1 long or 2 smaller rectangle loafs. Bake 50 minutes, or until a thermometer inserted in the middle reads 160 degrees.
7. Remove from the oven and rest for 10 minutes.
8. Meanwhile, when the meatloaf is almost ready, combine the cold beef broth, thyme and flour in a small saucepan and whisk well over medium heat until it comes to a boil, then simmer over medium-low heat until it thickens, stirring occasionally about 5 minutes.
9. Pour the pan drippings, if any into the gravy and continue to whisk another minute. Adjust salt and pepper to taste, as needed, then discard thyme.
10. Slice the loaf into 24 slices (if making 1, or 12 slices each if making this into 2 loaves) and serve hot with the gravy. Garnish with parsley if desired.

MUSHROOM KALE LASAGNA ROLLS

6

NUTRITION:
Calories: 258kcal, Carbohydrates: 30.5g, Protein: 11.5g, Fat: 8.4g, Saturated Fat: 6.5g, Cholesterol: 41mg, Sodium: 208mg, Fiber: 3g, Sugar: 2g

INGREDIENTS

- 10 9 oz dry lasagna noodles, cooked
- 2 1/2 cups marinara sauce
- 5 cups kale, stems removed, chopped fine
- 8 oz mushrooms, chopped fine
- 1 tsp olive oil
- 2 cloves garlic, chopped
- 15 oz part skim ricotta cheese
- 1/2 cup grated Parmesan cheese
- 1 egg, whisked
- salt and fresh pepper
- 3 oz 10 tbsp part-skim mozzarella cheese, shredded

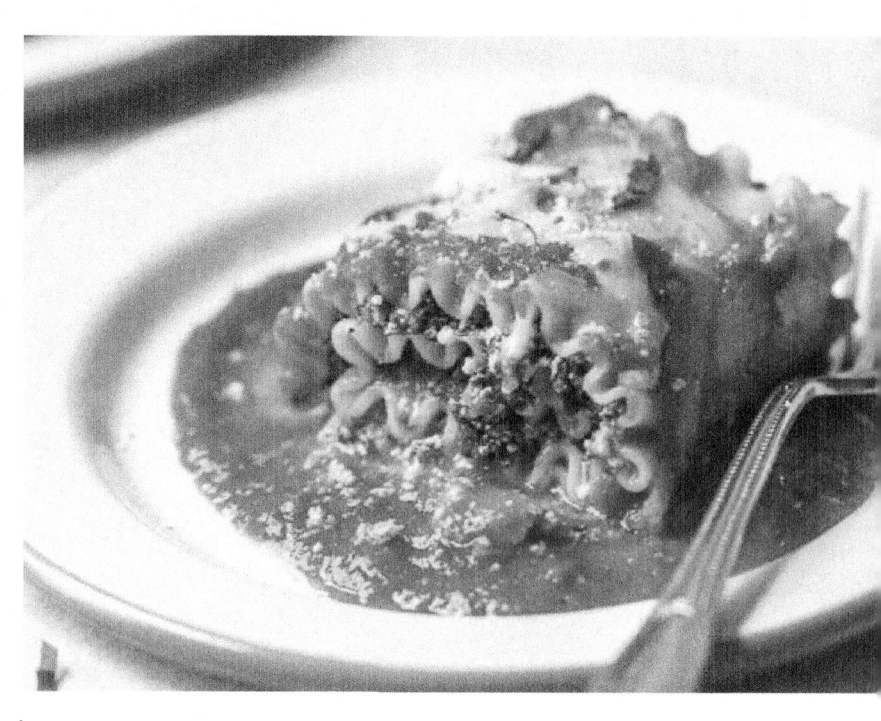

DIRECTION

1. Preheat oven to 350F.
2. Ladle about 1 cup sauce on the bottom of a 9 x 12 baking dish.
3. Place kale in a food processor and pulse a few times until chopped.
4. In a large skillet, heat oil over medium heat. Add garlic and sauté until golden, about a minute. Add kale, salt and pepper and sauté about 5 minutes.
5. Add mushrooms to the pan, cook until soft, an additional 5-6 minutes. Adjust salt and pepper, to taste.
6. Combine cooked kale, mushrooms, ricotta, Parmesan cheese, egg, salt and pepper in a medium bowl. Place a piece of wax paper on the counter and lay out cooked lasagna noodles. Make sure noodles are dry.
7. Take 1/3 cup of mushroom kale mixture and spread evenly over noodle. Roll carefully and place seam side down onto the baking dish. Repeat with remaining noodles.
8. Ladle 1 cup of sauce over the noodles in the baking dish and top each one with 1 tbsp mozzarella cheese. Put foil over baking dish and bake for 40 minutes, until cheese melts.
9. Makes 10 rolls. Serve with extra sauce on the side.

04
Appetizer

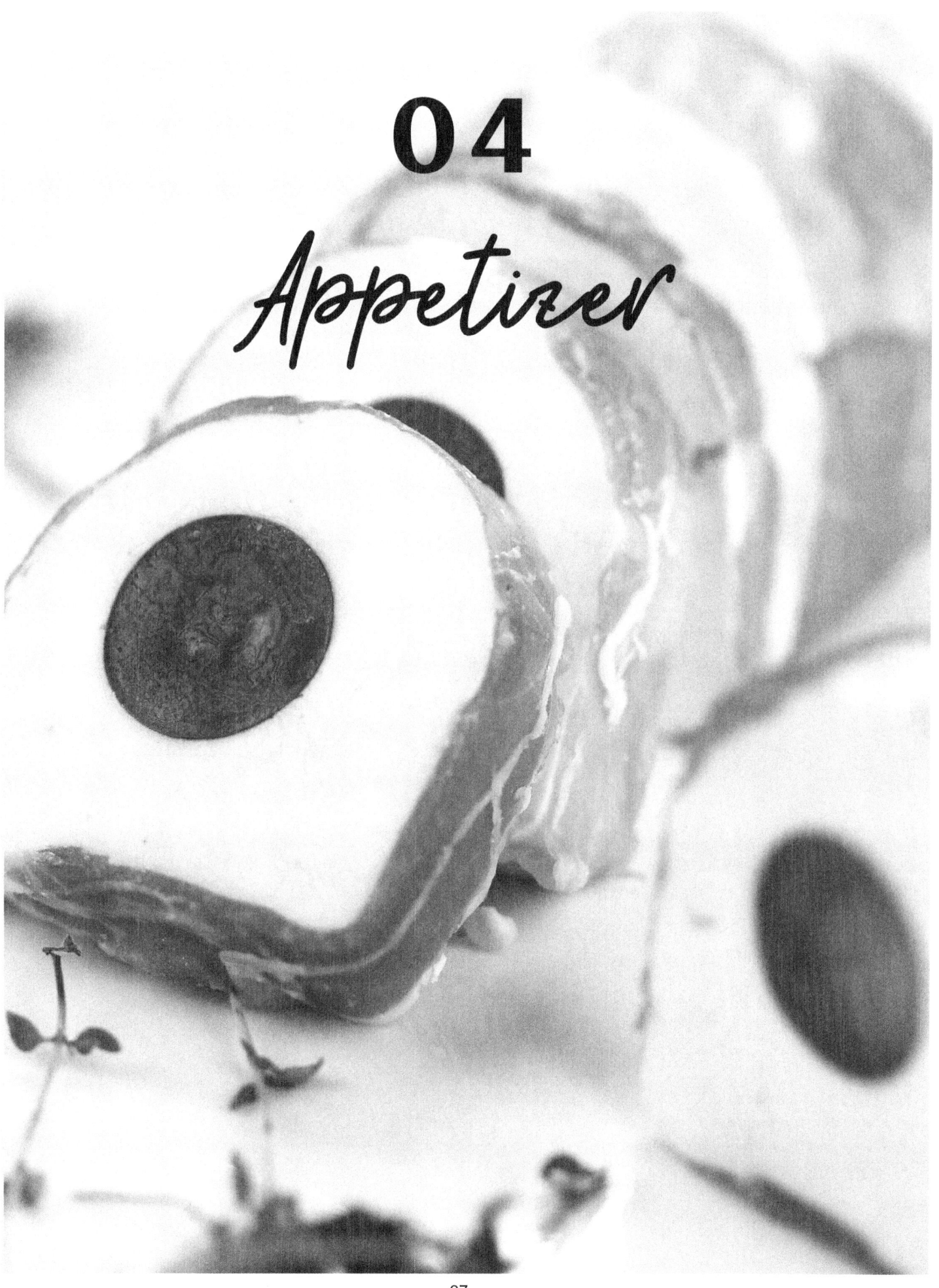

SHRIMP CEVICHE `1`

Calories: 147kcal, Carbohydrates: 7g, Protein: 24g, Fat: 2g, Saturated Fat: 1g, Cholesterol: 167mg, Sodium: 553mg, Fiber: 1g, Sugar: 2g

INGREDIENTS

- 1 pound fresh peeled and deveined shrimp, chopped (preferably wild)
- 1 cup fresh squeezed lime juice, from 6 to 9 limes
- 1/4 cup chopped red onion
- 1 1/2 teaspoons kosher salt
- 2/3 cup peeled and diced cucumber
- 1 to 2 jalapeño, stemmed and sliced into rings
- 1/4 cup chopped cilantro
- 1 scallions, chopped
- tortilla chips or plantain chips, for serving

DIRECTION

1. In a large bowl combine the shrimp, lime juice, red onion and salt.
2. Let it sit for 20 minutes, stirring occasionally until opaque.
3. Add the cucumbers, jalapeño, cilantro and scallion.
4. Serve right away with chips.

PICO DE GALLO SALSA `0`

Calories: 36.5kcal, Carbohydrates: 8g, Protein: 1g, Fat: 0.5g, Sodium: 13mg, Fiber: 1.5g, Sugar: 0.3g

INGREDIENTS

- 4 medium ripe tomatoes, chopped
- 1/2 cup finely chopped white onion
- 1-2 jalapeño or serrano pepper, seeded and finely chopped
- 1/4 cup finely chopped fresh cilantro leaves, no stems
- 2 tbsp fresh lime juice
- kosher salt and pepper, to taste
- 2 tbsp chopped red bell pepper, (optional)
- 1 clove garlic, minced (optional)

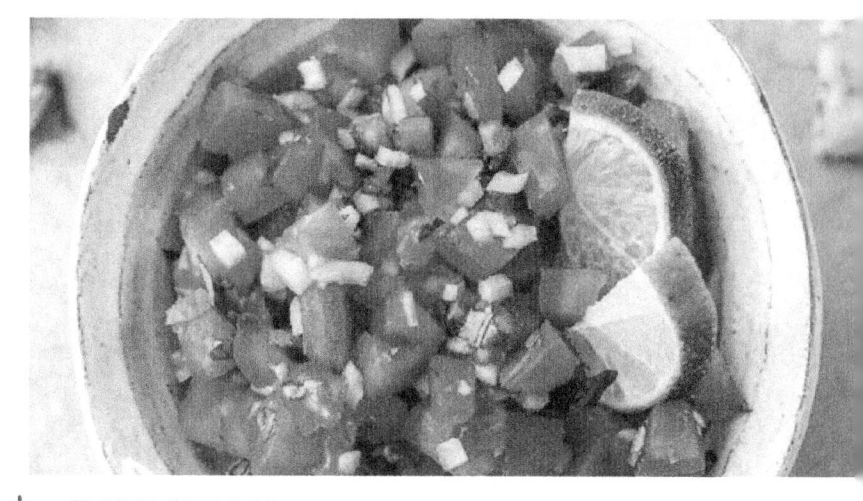

DIRECTION

1. In a bowl combine all ingredients.
2. Let it marinate in the refrigerator at least an hour for best results.

SPICY CRUNCHY TUNA TARTARE

5

Calories: 197.6kcal, Carbohydrates: 7.9g, Protein: 18.6g, Fat: 10.3g, Fiber: 3.1g

INGREDIENTS
- 8 oz sushi grade ahi tuna, finely chopped
- 2 tsp pure sesame oil, 1 tsp rice wine
- 2 tsp fresh lime juice
- 2 tsp soy sauce, or gluten-free tamari
- 1 tsp sriracha, or more to taste
- 2 tbsp chives, minced
- 2 tbsp panko crumbs, plain or gluten-free
- 1 ripe, firm hass avocado, diced
- 1 tsp black and white sesame seeds

DIRECTION
1. Combine sesame oil, rice wine, lime juice, soy sauce and sriracha in a medium bowl.
2. Poor over tuna and mix.
3. Add chives and gently combine tuna with diced avocado, refrigerate until ready to serve.
4. Add panko crumbs just before serving and top with sesame seeds.

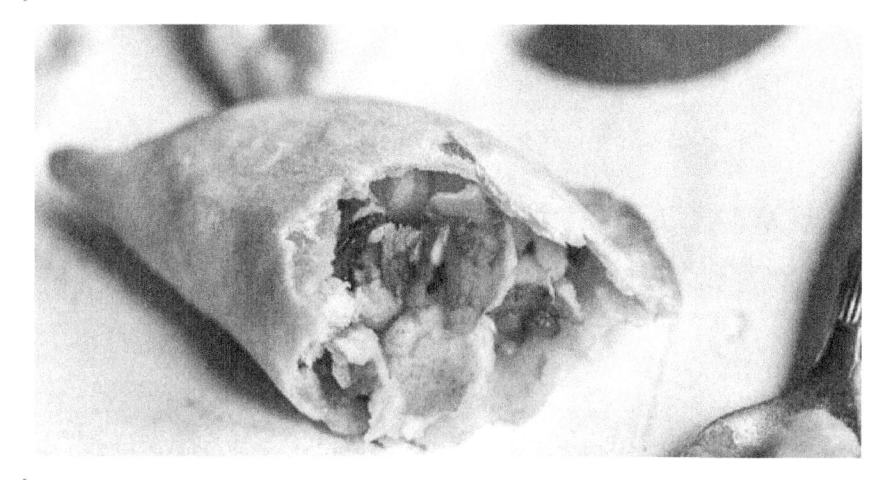

AIR FRYER LOBSTER JALAPENO EMPANADAS

5

Calories: 36.5kcal, Carbohydrates: 8g, Protein: 1g, Fat: 0.5g, Sodium: 13mg, Fiber: 1.5g, Sugar: 0.3g

INGREDIENTS
- 8 frozen empanada discs, thawed
- 1 teaspoon unsalted butter
- 2 tablespoons diced onion
- 1 jalapeno, minced
- 8 ounces roughly chopped raw lobster meat, I buy frozen claws from Crowd Cow
- 2 tablespoons chopped chives
- 1 large egg white, beaten
- 1 lime cut unto wedges, for serving

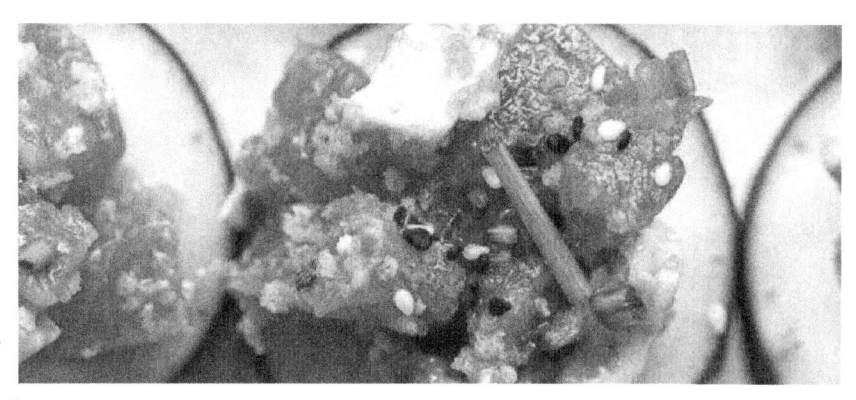

DIRECTION

To make the filling
1. Melt the butter in a heavy skillet over medium heat.
2. Add the onions and jalapeno and sauté until soft, about 2 to 3 minutes.
3. Add the lobster and cook 1 to 2 minutes until just opaque.
4. Remove from the heat and add the chives.
5. Quickly drain in a mesh sieve and set aside to cool.

To make the empanadas
1. Place the dough circles on a work surface.
2. Place about 2 tablespoons of lobster stuffing in the middle of a circle; brush the edges of the dough with the water or egg wash.
3. Fold the circle over itself, press the edges with your fingers or a fork to seal, and place on a work surface.
4. Repeat until all of the empanadas are filled. Brush tops with egg wash.
5. Spray the basket with oil to prevent sticking, transfer to the basket, in batches cook at 325F° for 8 minutes, turning half way.
6. Serve hot with lime wedges.

AIR FRYER BUFFALO CHICKEN ZUCCHINI SKINS 1

Calories: 80kcal, Carbohydrates: 3.5g, Protein: 9.5g, Fat: 3g, Saturated Fat: 1.5g, Cholesterol: 25.5mg, Sodium: 452.5mg, Fiber: 1g, Sugar: 2g

INGREDIENTS

- 2 large zucchini, about 9 ounces each
- olive oil spray
- 1/2 teaspoon salt, 1/4 teaspoon garlic powder
- 1/4 teaspoon paprika

Buffalo Chicken Stuffing:

- 7 ounce shredded skinless chicken breasts, from rotiserie chicken or make in slow cooker
- 1 ounces 1/3 less fat cream cheese, softened
- 1/4 cup Franks hot sauce, plus more for drizzling on top
- 4 teaspoons crumbled blue cheese or gorgonzola
- 1/4 cup light Blue Cheese or Ranch Dressing
- 2 tablespoons chopped scallions

DIRECTION

1. Combine the cream cheese and hot sauce together in a medium bowl until smooth. Add the chicken.
2. Cut zucchini in half lengthwise; then cut in half to give you 8 pieces. Scoop out the pulp on each piece, leaving a 1/4-inch shell on all sides (save pulp for another use).
3. Place zucchini skins on a work surface. Spray both sides with olive oil then season both sides with salt, then cut side with garlic powder and paprika.
4. Cook 350F in batches for 8 minutes, until tender-crisp. Place 3-4 tablespoons buffalo chicken inside each skin and top with 1/2 teaspoon cheese, dividing equally. Cook until cheese is melted, about 2 minutes longer. Serve right away each drizzled with 1/2 tablespoon blue cheese dressing topped with scallions for garnish. Serve hot.

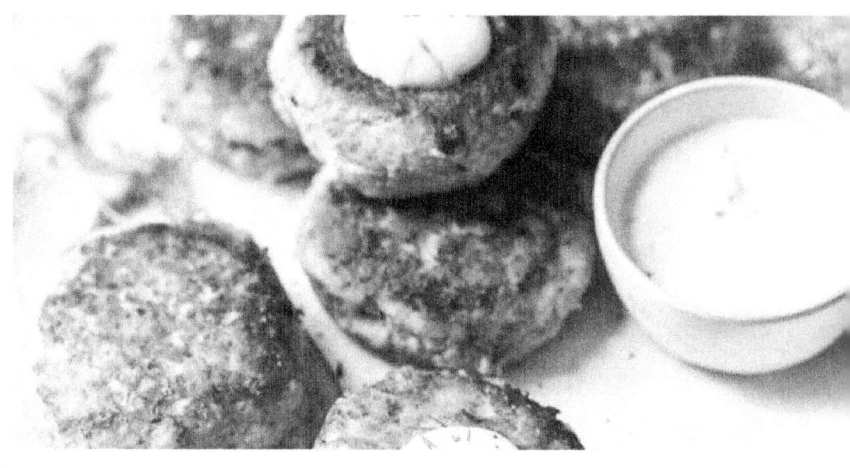

SALMON CROQUETTES WITH DILL SAUCE 3

Calories: 36.5kcal, Carbohydrates: 8g, Protein: 1g, Fat: 0.5g, Sodium: 13mg, Fiber: 1.5g, Sugar: 0.3g

INGREDIENTS

- For the sauce:
- 1 1/2 cups plain yogurt or light sour cream
- 1/4 cup Dijon mustard
- 6 sprigs fresh dill, chopped
- For the salmon:
- 4 cans, 7.5 ounces each unsalted salmon, packed in water
- 4 celery stalks, finely chopped
- 1 large white onion, finely chopped
- 4 large eggs, beaten
- 1/2 tablespoon salt
- black pepper, to taste
- 1 tablespoon olive oil

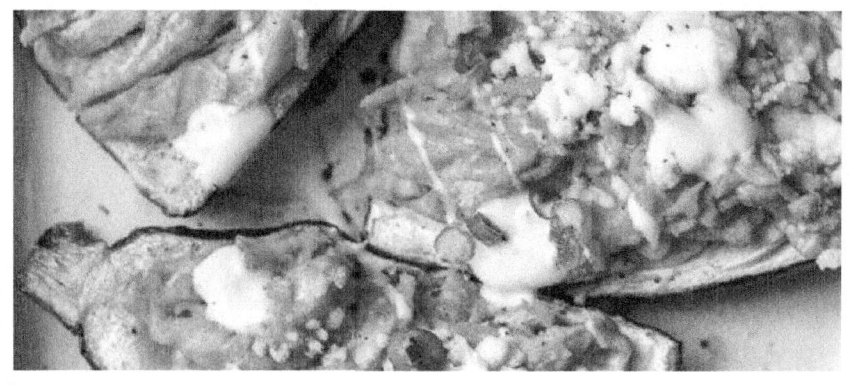

DIRECTION

1. Combine the dill sauce ingredients and set aside.
2. Drain the salmon, remove and discard the skin and bones.
3. Add it to a medium bowl with celery, onion, egg, salt and black pepper.
4. Form into 8 patties, pressing together so they hold, they will be delicate.
5. Heat a large skillet and add the oil, cook until browned on each side, about 5 minutes per side.
6. Serve with a dollop of the sauce on each patty and serve.

BABA GANOUSH

3

Calories: 140kcal, Carbohydrates: 15.5g, Protein: 2.5g, Fat: 9g, Saturated Fat: 1g Sodium: 743.5mg, Fiber: 4.5g, Sugar: 5g

INGREDIENTS

- 2 pounds eggplant, 2 medium or 1 large
- 3 tablespoons tahini paste, check label for GF
- 2 tbsp lemon juice
- 2 tbsp extra virgin olive oil
- 2 teaspoons kosher salt
- 1/4 teaspoon freshly ground black pepper
- 1 small garlic clove, minced fine

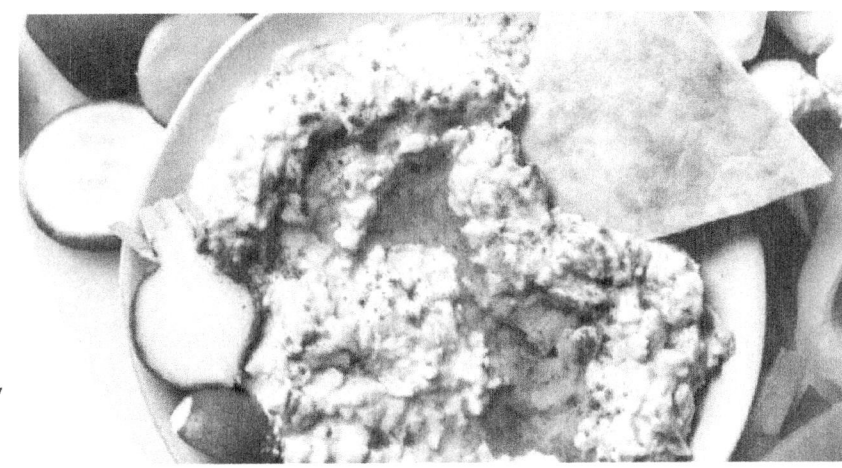

DIRECTION

1. Pierce the eggplant all over with a knife. Char the eggplant on the grill or in the broiler. If charbroiling, place eggplant on a foil-lined baking sheet under the broiler.
2. For the grill and broiler, cook for 20-25 minutes, turning every 5 minutes, until the eggplant is charred and blackened.
3. Let the eggplant cool. Then scoop the charred eggplant out of its skin and finely dice by hand or in a food processor. Discard the skin.
4. In a medium bowl, whisk together the tahini, lemon juice, olive oil, salt, pepper, and garlic.
5. Finely chop the eggplant, stir it into the tahini mixture, and season with more salt to taste.
6. Chill for at least one hour to let the flavors meld.

GRILLED CRAB LEGS

3

Calories: 144kcal, Protein: 31.5g, Fat: 1g, Cholesterol: 72mg, Sodium: 1400mg

INGREDIENTS

- 4 lbs frozen king, snow or dungeness crab legs, thawed and rinsed
- olive oil spray
- lemon wedges
- melted butter, optional for dipping

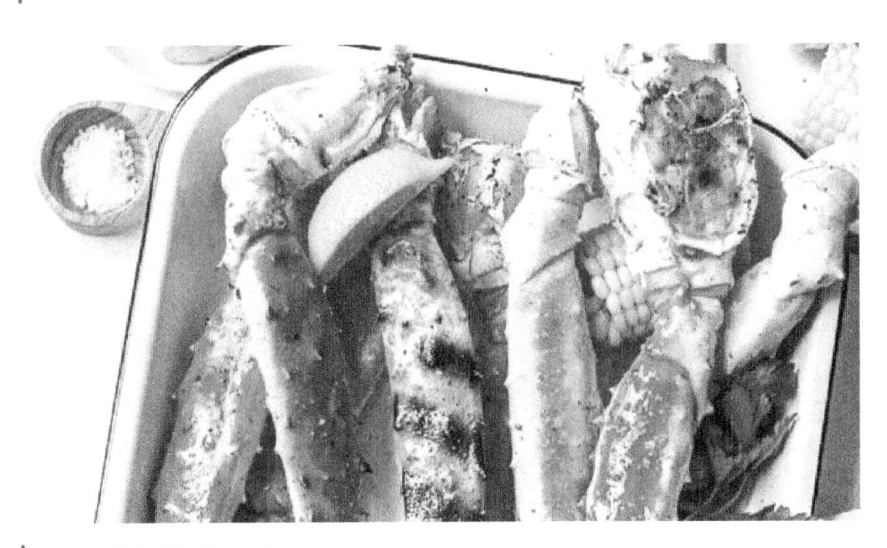

DIRECTION

1. Heat grill to medium-high.
2. Spritz crab legs all over with olive oil spray and place on hot grill.
3. Cover and cook about 7 minutes on each side, or until the meat in the center is heated through.
4. Use a sharp paring knife (and a mitt or glove to handle) and cut slits along the side so it's easy to pull the meat out.
5. Remove to plates and serve with lemon wedges and melted butter, if desired.

SHRIMP EGG ROLLS 2

Nutrition: Per Serving: 522 calories; protein 34.1g; carbohydrates 25.8g; dietary fiber 3.7g; sugars 2.2g; fat 31.9g; saturated fat 8.9g; cholesterol 93.2mg

INGREDIENTS

- 1 tablespoon toasted sesame oil
- 1 teaspoon grated ginger
- 3 garlic cloves, minced
- 2 large scallions, chopped
- 3 cups chopped green cabbage
- 1/2 cups shredded carrots
- 2 tablespoons reduced sodium soy sauce
- 1/2 tablespoon unseasoned rice vinegar
- 1/2 pound large peeled raw shrimp, chopped
- 6 egg roll wrappers
- Olive oil spray
- Sweet chili sauce, duck sauce or spicy mustard, for dipping (optional)

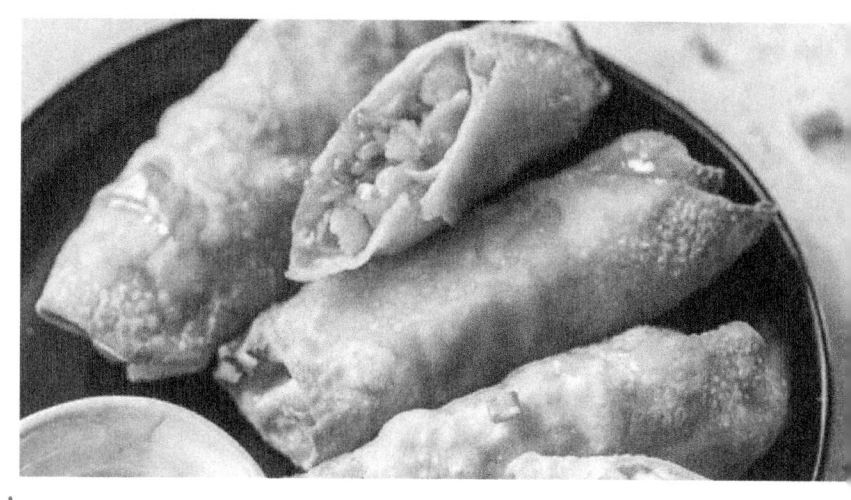

DIRECTION

1. In a large skillet, heat sesame oil over medium-high heat. Add the shrimp and sauté, until shrimp is almost cooked through, 1 to 2 minutes.
2. Add ginger, garlic and scallions. Sauté until fragrant, about 30 seconds. Add cabbage and carrots, soy sauce and vinegar.
3. Cook on high heat until vegetables are tender crisp, about 2 to 3 minutes. Transfer to a colander to drain and let cool.
4. One at a time, place egg roll wrapper on a clean surface, points facing top and bottom like a diamond. Spoon a 1/3 cup mixture onto the bottom third of the wrapper.
5. Dip your finger in a small bowl of water and run it along the edges of the wrapper. Lift the point nearest you and wrap it around the filling.
6. Fold the left and right corners in toward the center and continue to roll into a tight cylinder. Set aside and repeat with remaining wrappers and filling.
7. Spray all sides of the egg rolls with oil using your fingers to evenly coat.
8. In batches, cook 370F for 5 to 7 minutes, turning halfway through until golden brown.
9. Serve immediately, with dipping sauce on the side, if desired.

MARGARITA PIZZA

6

Calories: 236kcal, Carbohydrates: 27g, Protein: 15g, Fat: 6.5g, Saturated Fat: 3.5g Cholesterol: 23.5mg, Sodium: 636mg, Fiber: 1g, Sugar: 3.5g

INGREDIENTS

- 1 cup all purpose or white whole wheat flour*, (5 oz) plus more for dusting
- 1 1/2 teaspoons baking powder
- 1/2 teaspoon kosher salt
- 1 cup 0% Stonyfield Greek yogurt, not regular, drained if there's any liquid
- Sauce
- 1/3 cup canned san marzano tomatoes, crushed by hand
- 1 small garlic clove, minced
- 1/4 teaspoon kosher salt
- pinch dried oregano
- fresh black pepper to taste
- 4 ounces fresh mozzarella cheese, sliced thin and torn by hand
- fresh basil, torn for topping
- extra virgin olive oil, optional for drizzling

DIRECTION

1. In a medium bowl combine the flour, baking powder and salt and whisk well.
2. Add the yogurt and mix with a fork or spatula until well combined, it will look like small crumbles.
3. Lightly dust flour on a work surface and remove dough from the bowl, knead the dough a few times until dough is tacky, but not sticky, about 20 turns (it should not leave dough on your hand when you pull away).
4. Preheat oven to 450F. I like to use a pizza stone, and preheat the stone in the oven as well. If using a round pizza pan or sheet pan, spray with oil.
5. Sprinkle a work surface and rolling pin with a little flour and roll the dough out into a large thin round or oval (or you can make 2 smaller pies).
6. Lay the dough out onto the oiled nonstick pizza dish or sheet pan.
7. Spread the sauce over the crust. Top with cheese and place the pan on the pizza stone, bake 10 to 12 minutes or until the cheese is bubbly and the crust is cooked through.
8. Transfer to a cutting board, top with basil and drizzle with olive oil, if desired. Slice the pie into 8 slices.

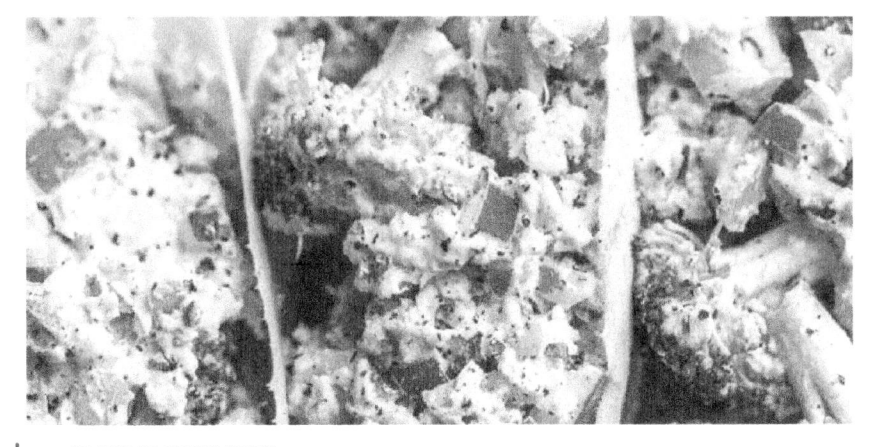

TUNA SALAD WRAPS

4

Calories: 160kcal, Carbohydrates: 4.5g, Protein: 22g, Fat: 6g, Saturated Fat: 1g, Cholesterol: 30mg, Sodium: 415mg, Fiber: 1g, Sugar: 1g

INGREDIENTS

- 1 5 ounce can light tuna in water, drained
- 1/4 cup chopped celery, 1/4 cup chopped red onion, 1/4 cup broccoli florets
- 2 tbsp Hellmann's light mayonnaise, regular for Keto
- 1 tsp red wine vinegar
- 1 head endive, leaves separated

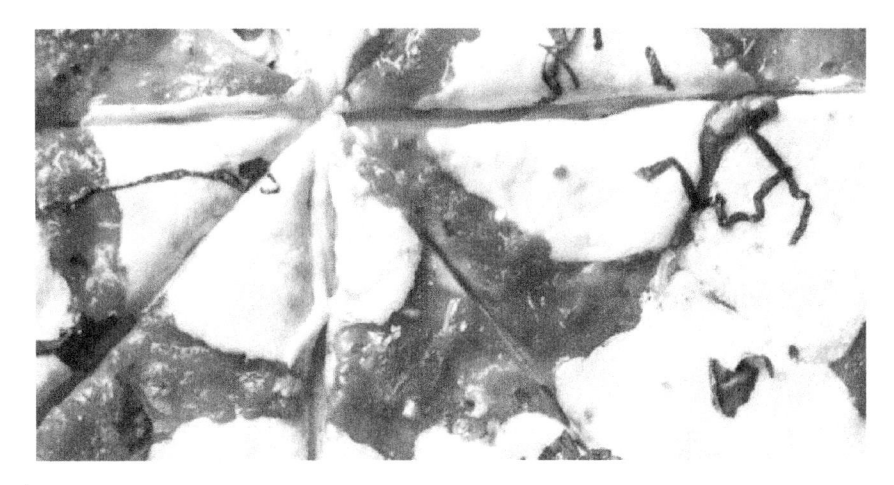

DIRECTION

1. Combine all the tuna salad ingredients and spoon into endive leaves.

PIZZA SAUSAGE ROLLS

8

Nutrition: Per Serving: 522 calories; protein 34.1g; carbohydrates 25.8g; dietary fiber 3.7g; sugars 2.2g; fat 31.9g; saturated fat 8.9g; cholesterol 93.2mg

INGREDIENTS

- For bagel dough:
- 1 cup unbleached all-purpose flour, plus more for dusting, (5 oz in weight) use cup4cup for GF*
- 2 teaspoons baking powder
- 3/4 teaspoon kosher salt
- 1 cup non-fat Greek yogurt, (should be thick) I recommend Stonyfield
- 1 egg white, beaten (whole egg works fine too)
- sesame seeds, for topping (optional)
- For filling:
- 2 raw chicken Italian sausage links, 3 oz total (halved lengthwise) I like Premio
- 4 slices provolone or mozzarella cheese
- 8 teaspoons pizza sauce or marinara
- marinara sauce, for serving (optional)

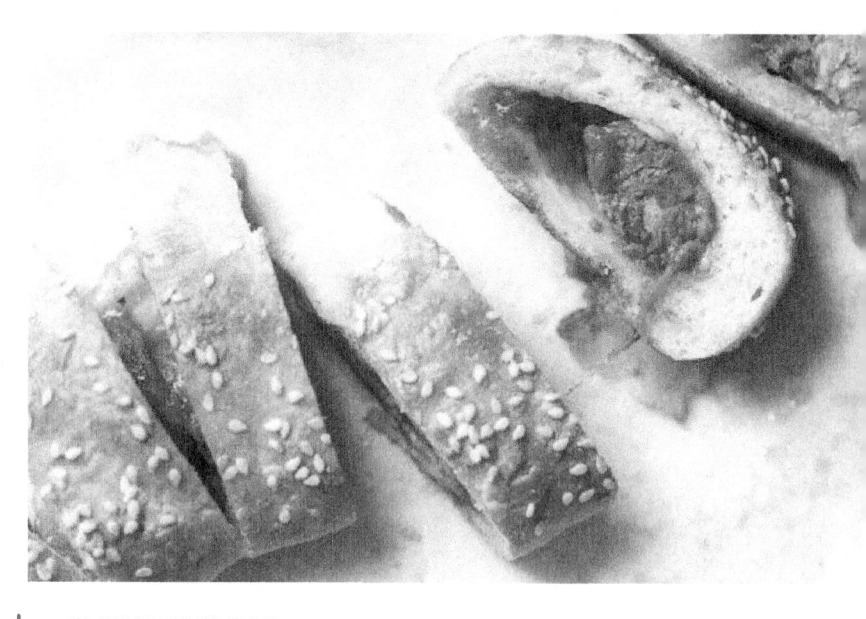

DIRECTION

1. Preheat oven to 400 degrees F. Place parchment paper or a silpat on a baking sheet. If using parchment paper, spray with oil to avoid sticking.
2. In a medium bowl combine the flour, baking powder and salt and whisk well.
3. Add the yogurt and mix with a fork or spatula until well combined (it will be sticky and look like small crumbles).
4. Lightly dust flour on a work surface and remove dough from the bowl, knead the dough a few times until dough is tacky, but not sticky, about 15 turns (it should not leave dough on your hand when you pull away). If it's too sticky, add a few extra sprinkles of flour.
5. Divide in 4 equal balls.
6. Working with 1 ball at a time, lightly dust a rolling pin and a work surface and roll dough into a 5 ½" circle, about ¼" thick.
7. Spread 2 teaspoons pizza sauce down the middle of the circle, leaving about 1/2" border.
8. Lay 1 slice of cheese in the middle of the circle then top with 1/2 sausage link.
9. Carefully bring both sides of the dough up, wrap one side around the sausage then the other.
10. Press dough together so it's sealed around the sausage and place it on the prepared sheet pan seam side-down.
11. Repeat with remaining dough, sauce, cheese and sausage.
12. Brush each with egg wash, top with sesame seeds, if using, and bake for 25-30 minutes.
13. Allow to cool for 5 minutes then slice into 6 pieces and serve.

WHIPPED RICOTTA TOAST WITH ROASTED GARLIC, TOMATOES AND SHALLOTS

7

Calories: 256kcal, Carbohydrates: 35g, Protein: 12g, Fat: 7.5g, Saturated Fat: 3g, Cholesterol: 15mg, Sodium: 586mg, Fiber: 2.5g, Sugar: 4g

INGREDIENTS

- 1 medium head garlic
- 3 teaspoons olive oil
- Kosher salt
- Freshly ground black pepper
- 1 dry pint grape tomatoes, halved
- 1 medium shallot, cut into ¼-inch slices
- 8- ounces French baguette
- Olive oil spray
- 1 cup part skim milk ricotta
- ¼ cup chopped basil, for garnish
- Crushed red pepper flakes, for garnish (optional)

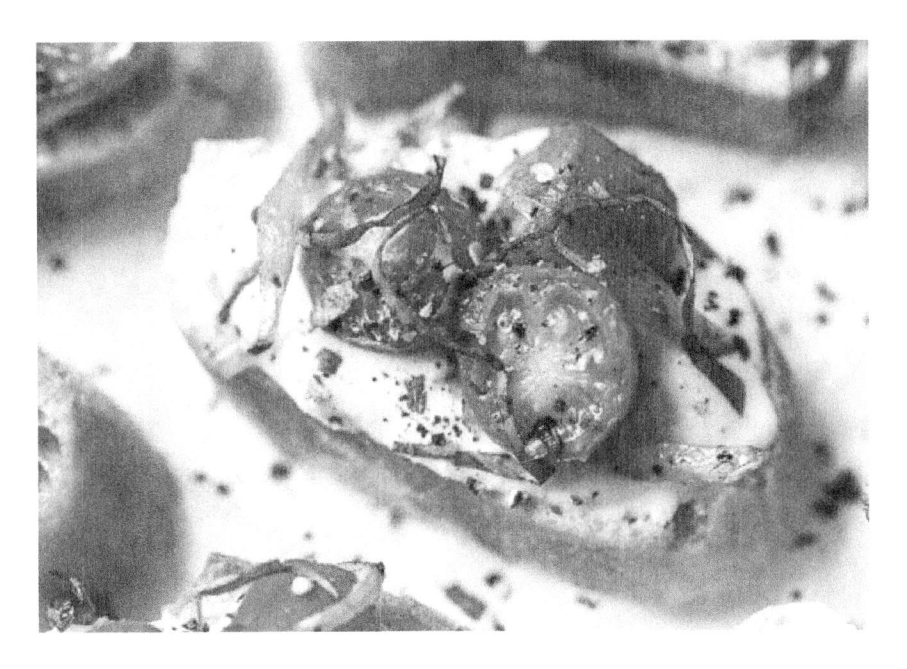

DIRECTION

1. Preheat oven to 400 degrees F.
2. Cut just the top of the head of garlic off, leaving cloves intact and exposed. Drizzle with 1 teaspoon oil, wrap tightly in aluminum foil, place on medium sheet pan and roast for 25 minutes.
3. In a medium bowl, combine the tomatoes, shallots, remaining 2 teaspoons oil, ½ teaspoon salt and pepper, to taste. Toss to coat. Transfer to a sheet pan lined with parchment.
4. After garlic has roasted for 25 minutes, leave it in the oven then add the sheet pan with the tomatoes and shallots and roast for 20 minutes.
5. Meanwhile, cut bread into 20 (½-inch) slices.
6. Remove both sheet pans from the oven. Turn the oven off, take wrapped garlic off sheet pan and allow to cool for 5 minutes.
7. Lay bread slices in an even layer on the sheet pan, spray lightly with olive oil and place the sheet pan in the oven to allow bread to toast while you whip the ricotta.
8. Unwrap the garlic and carefully squeeze or scoop cloves into a food processor fitted with metal blade. Add the ricotta, ¼ teaspoon salt and pepper, to taste then process for 30 seconds. Scrap sides with a spatula and pulse 2-3 times to thoroughly combine.
9. Remove bread from oven and assemble toast.
10. To assemble toast:
11. Scoop 1 tablespoon of whipped ricotta onto each piece of bread. Evenly distribute tomatoes and shallots on to toasts.
12. Top each with basil, a pinch of salt and red pepper flakes, if using. Serve immediately.

ASPARAGUS AND FETA TARTLET WITH PHYLLO CRUST `2`

Calories: 91kcal, Carbohydrates: 7.5g, Protein: 4.5g, Fat: 5g, Saturated Fat: 2.5g, Cholesterol: 73.5mg, Sodium: 170mg, Fiber: 0.5g, Sugar: 1.5g

INGREDIENTS

- 12 medium asparagus, about 4 ounces
- 2 olive oil spray, divided, plus
- 2 garlic cloves, finely chopped
- 1 tablespoon lemon juice
- 1/4 teaspoon salt
- 1/4 teaspoon freshly ground black pepper
- 1 1/3 ounces feta cheese, crumbled
- 6 tablespoons half and half
- 1 large egg
- 1 tablespoon chopped fresh dill
- 4 phyllo sheets

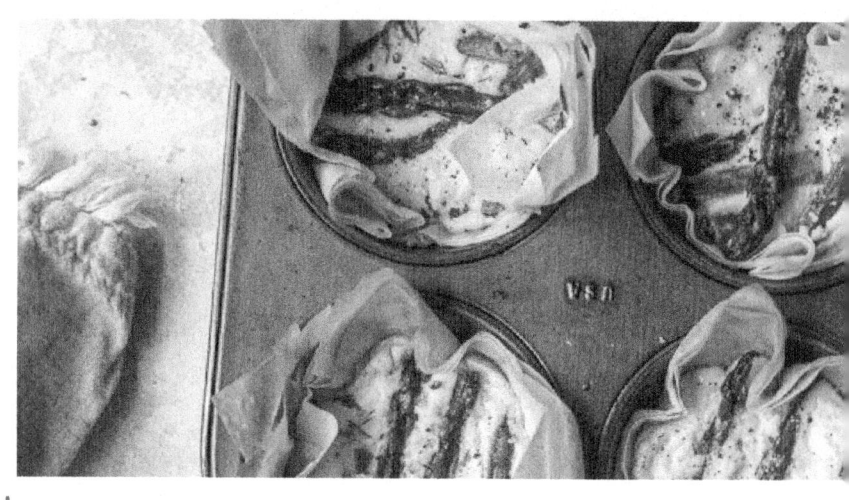

DIRECTION

1. Heat oven to 350° F. Lightly spray 6 cups in a muffin tin with olive oil spray.
2. Snap off and discard the woody end of the asparagus.
3. Cut 1 1/2-inch long pieces from the tip end. Cut the remaining parts of the stalks into 1-inch pieces.
4. Spray nonstick pan with olive oil spray over medium high heat. Add asparagus and garlic and sauté, stirring, for 2 minutes.
5. Stir in the lemon juice and 1 tablespoon water. Reduce heat to low, cover and cook for 1 minute more.
6. Remove asparagus pieces to a plate using a slotted spoon and reserve the pan juices and garlic.
7. Place a phyllo sheet on a clean work surface, lightly spray with oil and top with another phyllo sheet. Repeat with two more sheets and oil.
8. Cut the phyllo into 4-inch squares. Fit one square each in the prepared muffin cups. .
9. Evenly distribute the 1-inch asparagus pieces and feta among the muffin cups.
10. Whisk half and half, egg, dill, and reserved pan juices together. Evenly divide among the phyllo cups (about 3 1/2 tablespoons in each).
11. Place two asparagus tips on each cup and bake for for 30 minutes until custard is set and phyllo is golden.

Printed in Great Britain
by Amazon